CALORIE CARBOHYDRATE COUNTER

1988 Edition

P.S.I. & Associates, Inc.
10481 S.W. 123rd Street
Miami, Florida 33176

INTRODUCTION

The *Calorie and Carbohydrate Counter* is a compact, yet complete, list of several thousand basic foods and brand-name products with their caloric and carbohydrate content.

The calorie intake of your diet in relation to the amount of energy you expend determines whether you maintain, gain, or lose weight. Individuals who watch their weight, for various health reasons, have taken to counting the calories in their diet.

To learn how many calories you are consuming each day, keep a record of your total caloric intake of food and beverages for one week. Weigh yourself at the beginning and at the end of that week. If your weight is the same at the end of the week as it was in the beginning, then the total number of calories for that week is your *approximate* maintenance level. *Approximate* is emphasized here because your level of activity may vary, thereby varying the number of calories your body burns. To lose weight, you must reduce your weekly caloric intake below this maintenance level. To gain weight, you must increase your caloric intake above this maintenance level.

Some dieticians are also directing attention to the carbohydrate content of the diet in relation to weight control. It is for those individuals who are counting their carbohydrates, along with their calories, that this information is included in the chart.

Calories

A calorie is a unit used to measure quantities of heat energy. The large calorie is used to measure the amount of heat required to raise the temperature of one kilogram of water one degree centigrade.

If the caloric content of your diet

exceeds the amount that your body needs, the extra calories will be stored as fat. 3500 calories is equal to one pound of fat. So, to gain one pound, you must add 3500 calories to your maintenance level. Conversely, you must subtract 3500 calories from your maintenance level to lose one pound.

Carbohydrates

Carbohydrates are composed of carbon, hydrogen, and oxygen. Sugar, starch, and cellulose are a few types of carbohydrates. All ordinary plants are primarily carbohydrates. These compounds are present in smaller quantities in animals. Carbohydrates are fuel for the body. Any excess amounts of carbohydrates in our diet can be stored in the body and used when quick energy is needed. Otherwise, they are converted to body fat. The values given in this chart are total carbohydrates, by difference.

Remember that protein, fat, minerals and vitamins are important when planning your diet. Eat a variety of foods from the basic food groups; meat, fish and poultry; vegetables and fruits; breads and cereals; and milk, to obtain the essential nutrients your body requires. Individuals who count their calories should be able to find a variety of appetizing foods in keeping with their specific diet.

How To Use This Dictionary

Foods are listed alphabetically by the name of the basic food or by the brand name. All entries are listed by groups of foods. For example, all cereals are grouped together. So, if you are looking for Oatmeal, you look first under Cereals, then under O in alphabetical order. Some entries are further broken down into sub-groups and are indented. For example, to find *Borden* Pimentoflavored unwhipped Cream Cheese, first look under Cheese, then under Cream Cheese, Flavored, Unwhipped. Indented below this entry in alphabetical order you find: Pimento *(Borden)*.

Similarly, to find *Vita* Bismark Herring in Cream Sauce, first look under Fish, then under Herring, Bismark. Indented below this entry in alphabetical order you find: In cream sauce *(Vita)*.

Under the main headings, it was not always possible to follow an alphabetical arrangement. The first entries under most basic foods are brand names of those foods, followed by an alphabetical listing of sub-groups. This basic format, with adaptations where necessary, was followed throughout the book.

All company names appear in italics in parentheses at the end of each entry. Figures from the United States Department of Agriculture are averages from several manufacturers and are used where specific brand names are not available.

Measures or Quantities Used

It is important to note the Measure or Quantity column. Where possible, common household measures are used. However, some measures listed are those commonly purchased in the store, such as 1 pound of beef or a 12½-oz. frozen dinner. To determine the caloric and carbohydrate count for each person served, divide these quantities given by the number of servings used. Also, any ingredients added in preparing the foods must be taken into account when recording your caloric and carbohydrate intake.

To keep an accurate account of the calories and carbohydrates in your diet, you also must be as accurate about the size of portions you use. Weigh your foods until you can visually gauge the weight. Keep in mind, as the weight of foods increases, so does the caloric and carbohydrate content. Also, remember that ounces by weight may be different from fluid ounces or fractions of a cup. Ounces in the chart are ounces by weight unless otherwise specified. Volume measure may vary depending on how tightly foods are packed into the cup. The weights of foods also vary when weighed with and without liquid.

In the Measure or Quantity column, such phrases as "weighed with bone" or "weighed with seeds" apply to the foods as you buy them in the store. The caloric and carbohydrate content as shown are only for the amount of edible food after you discard the inedible part.

Abbreviations and Symbols Used in this Dictionary

cu. — cubic
diam. — diameter
fl. — fluid
gr. — gram
in. — inch
lb. — pound
med. — medium
oz. — ounce
pkg. — package
tbsp. — tablespoon
tsp. — teaspoon
& — and
% — percent
x — by
* — Prepared as pkg. directs

(USDA) — United States Department of Agriculture

Blank space in columns — no available data

Weights and Measures

1 pound = 16 ounces

1 ounce = 28.349 grams

1 gallon = 4 quarts

1 quart = 2 pints = 4 cups

1 cup = 8 fluid ounces = ½ pint = 16 tablespoons

2 tablespoons = 1 fluid ounce

1 tablespoon = 3 teaspoons

1 inch = 2.540 centimeters

1 cubic inch = 16.387 cubic centimeters

Food Groups

Appetizers
Baby Food
Beverages — Non-Alcoholic
Beverages — Alcoholic
Breads
Cakes
Cake Needs
Candy — Noncommercial
Candy — Commercial
Candy — Dietetic
Cereals
Cheese
Cheese Spread
Cheese Dips
Cheese Fondue
Cheese Soufflé
Chewing Gum
Chinese Food
Chinese Dinner
Condiments
Cookies
Cookies — Dietetic
Cookie Mixes
Crackers, Puffs, Chips
Desserts

Eggs
Fats, Oils
Fish
Flavorings, Seasonings
Frozen Dinners
Fruits
Gelatin
Grain Products
Gravy
Ice Cream
Jellies and Preserves
Meat
Meats — Luncheon
Milk and Milk Products
Yoghurt
Nuts
Pancakes and Waffles
Pies and Pastry, Fillings, Crusts
Poultry
Salad Dressings and Mixes
Sandwich Spreads
Sauces and Sauce Mixes
Soups
Soup Mix
Sugars, Sweets, Syrups, Icings
Vegetables

Food and Description	Measure or Quantity	Calories	Carbo-hydrates (grams)
APPETIZERS			
Anchovy Paste, Canned			
(Crosse & Blackwell)	1 tbsp.	20	1.0
Caviar, Sturgeon,			
Dressed (USDA)	1 oz.	90	1.4
Whole eggs,	1 oz.	74	.9
Whole eggs (USDA)	1 tbsp.	42	.5
Cheese Puff, Frozen (Durkee)	1 piece	59	2.9
Dip Mix, Bacon-onion			
(Fritos)	1 pkg.	47	7.2
Blue cheese (Fritos)	1 pkg.	48	8.1
Green onion (Fritos)	1 pkg.	49	10.8
(Lawry's)	1 pkg.	50	10.6
Guacamole (Lawry's)	1 pkg.	60	5.5
Toasted onion (Fritos)	1 pkg.	47	10.0
(Lawry's)	1 pkg.	48	9.8
Taco (Fritos)	1 pkg.	43	10.0
Garlic Spread, (Lawry's)	1 tbsp.	79	1.2
Liverwurst, Spread,			
Canned (Underwood)	1 tbsp.	45	.5
Lobster, Paste, Canned			
(USDA)	1 oz.	51	.4
Meatball, Cocktail (Cresca)	1 meatball	10	
Oysters, Smoked, Japanese			
baby (Cresca)	3⅔-oz. can	222	
Pate, Canned, Swiss Parfait			
with truffles or herbs			
(Cresca)	1 oz.	73	
Canned, Liver (Hormel)	1 oz.	78	1.1
Canned, De foie gras			
(USDA)	1 oz.	131	1.4
Shrimp, Paste, Canned			
(USDA)	1 oz.	51	.4
Cocktail (Sau-Sea)	4-oz. jar	107	20.6
Cocktail (Sea Snack)	4-oz. jar	110	14.8
Puff, Frozen (Durkee)	1 piece	44	3.0
BABY FOOD			
Apple, Apple & apricot,			

Food and Description	Measure or Quantity	Calories	Carbo- hydrates (grams)
Junior (*Beech-Nut*)	7¾ oz.	212	51.2
Strained (*Beech-Nut*)	4¾ oz.	123	29.7
Apple Betty, Junior (*Beech-Nut*)	7¾ oz.	234	55.2
Strained (*Beech-Nut*)	4¾ oz.	147	34.8
Apple & cranberry, Junior (*Heinz*)	7¾ oz.	191	46.6
Strained (*Heinz*)	4¾ oz.	124	30.7
Apple & honey, Junior (*Heinz*)	7½ oz.	155	36.9
With tapioca, Strained (*Heinz*)	4½ oz.	89	21.8
Apple juice, Strained (*Beech-Nut*)	4-1/5 fl. oz. (4.4 oz.)	57	14.4
(*Gerber*)	4-1/5 fl. oz. (4.6 oz.)	65	16.0
(*Heinz*)	4½ fl. oz.	88	21.7
Apple-apricot juice, Strained (*Heinz*)	4½ fl. oz.	92	22.4
Apple-cherry juice, Strained (*Beech-Nut*)	4-1/5 fl. oz. (4.4 oz.)	74	18.4
Strained (*Gerber*)	4-1/5 fl. oz. (4.6 oz.)	59	14.2
Strained (*Heinz*)	4½ fl. oz.	86	21.1
Apple-grape juice, Strained (*Beech-Nut*)	4⅛ fl. oz. (4.4 oz.)	81	20.1
Strained (*Heinz*)	4½ fl. oz.	89	22.3
Apple-pineapple juice, Strained (*Heinz*)	4½ fl. oz.	92	22.5
Apple-prune juice, Strained (*Heinz*)	4½ fl. oz.	89	22.0
Apple & pear, Junior (*Heinz*)	7¾ oz.	180	43.7
Strained (*Heinz*)	4½ oz.	108	26.4
Apple pie, Junior (*Heinz*)	7¾ oz.	219	49.5
Strained (*Heinz*)	4¾ oz.	133	30.0

Food and Description	Measure or Quantity	Calories	Carbohydrates (grams)
Apple-prune & honey,			
Junior *(Heinz)*	7½ oz.	181	43.8
With tapioca, Strained,			
Junior *(Heinz)*	4½ oz.	107	25.4
Dutch apple dessert,			
Junior *(Gerber)*	7-8/10 oz.	204	47.8
Strained *(Gerber)*	4-7/10 oz.	124	28.5
Applesauce, Junior			
(Beech-Nut)	7¾ oz.	197	47.7
Junior *(Gerber)*	7-8/10 oz.	179	44.6
Junior *(Heinz)*	7¾ oz.	182	44.7
Strained *(Beech-Nut)*	4¾ oz.	121	29.5
Strained *(Gerber)*	4-7/10 oz.	109	27.4
Strained *(Heinz)*	4½ oz.	98	24.0
Applesauce & apricots,			
Junior *(Gerber)*	7-8/10 oz.	192	47.0
Junior *(Heinz)*	7¾ oz.	174	41.6
Strained *(Gerber)*	4-7/10 oz.	116	29.2
Strained *(Heinz)*	4¾ oz.	98	23.8
Applesauce & cherries,			
Junior *(Beech-Nut)*	7¾ oz.	206	48.8
Strained *(Beech-Nut)*	4¾ oz.	127	29.3
Applesauce & pineapple,			
Junior *(Gerber)*	7-8/10 oz.	162	41.7
Strained *(Gerber)*	4-7/10 oz.	106	26.4
Applesauce & raspberries,			
Junior *(Beech-Nut)*	7¾ oz.	243	57.8
Strained *(Beech-Nut)*	4¾ oz.	143	34.6
Apricot, With tapioca,			
Junior *(Beech-Nut)*	7¾ oz.	188	45.3
Junior *(Gerber)*	7-8/10 oz.	178	44.1
Junior *(Heinz)*	7¾ oz.	224	55.0
Strained *(Beech-Nut)*	4¾ oz.	103	25.1
Strained *(Gerber)*	4-7/10 oz.	107	26.4
Strained *(Heinz)*	4¾ oz.	141	33.3
Banana, Strained *(Heinz)*	4½ oz.	105	25.0
Dessert, Junior			
(Beech-Nut)	7¾ oz.	204	49.7
Pie, Junior *(Heinz)*	7¾ oz.	207	45.0

Food and Description	Measure or Quantity	Cal-ories	Carbo-hydrates (grams)
Strained (*Heinz*)	4¾ oz.	116	25.0
Banana & Pineapple,			
Junior (*Heinz*)	7¾ oz.	167	40.6
Strained (*Heinz*)	4¾ oz.	102	25.0
With tapioca, Junior			
(*Beech-Nut*)	7¾ oz.	204	49.9
Junior (*Gerber*)	7-8/10 oz.	181	44.6
Strained (*Beech-Nut*)	4¾ oz.	129	30.2
Strained (*Gerber*)	4-7/10 oz.	113	27.4
Pudding, Junior (*Gerber*)	7-8/10 oz.	210	48.2
With tapioca, Strained			
(*Beech-Nut*)	4¾ oz.	119	28.9
Strained (*Gerber*)	4-7/10 oz.	113	27.4
Bean, green, Junior			
(*Beech-Nut*)	7¼ oz.	62	12.5
Strained (*Beech-Nut*)	4½ oz.	40	7.8
Strained (*Gerber*)	4½ oz.	36	8.5
Strained (*Heinz*)	4½ oz.	37	6.4
Creamed with bacon,			
Junior (*Gerber*)	7½ oz.	141	19.0
In butter sauce, Junior			
(*Beech-Nut*)	7¼ oz.	94	16.8
Strained (*Beech-Nut*)	4½ oz.	58	10.2
With potatoes & ham			
casserole, Toddler			
(*Gerber*)	6-1/5 oz.	139	17.8
Beef, Junior (*Beech-Nut*)	3½ oz.	87	.3
Junior (*Gerber*)	3½ oz.	95	0
Strained (*Beech-Nut*)	3½ oz.	101	0
Beef & beef broth,			
Junior (*Heinz*)	3½ oz.	99	0
Strained (*Heinz*)	3½ oz.	92	0
Strained (*Gerber*)	3½ oz.	85	.7
Beef dinner, Junior			
(*Beech-Nut*)	4½ oz.	120	7.3
Strained (*Beech-Nut*)	4½ oz.	134	7.7
Beef dinner & noodles,			
Junior (*Beech-Nut*)	7½ oz.	138	15.7
Junior (*Gerber*)	7½ oz.	107	16.7

Food and Description	Measure or Quantity	Calories	Carbo-hydrates (grams)
Strained (Beech-Nut)	4½ oz.	79	9.4
Strained (Gerber)	4½ oz.	61	9.6
Strained (Heinz)	4½ oz.	59	9.3
With vegetables, Junior (Gerber)	4½ oz.	105	7.9
Strained (Gerber)	4½ oz.	104	8.0
Strained (Heinz)	4¾ oz.	109	7.1
With vegetables & cereal, Junior (Heinz)	4¾ oz.	110	5.8
Beef lasagna, Toddler (Gerber)	6-1/5 oz.	135	17.2
Beef liver, Strained (Gerber)	3½ oz.	92	2.0
Beef liver soup, Strained (Heinz)	4½ oz.	57	8.1
Beef stew, Toddler (Gerber)	6-1/5 oz.	120	15.2
Beet, Strained (Gerber)	4½ oz.	48	11.0
Strained (Heinz)	4½ oz.	60	12.7
Blueberry, Blueberry buckle, Junior (Gerber)	7-8/10 oz.	185	45.7
Strained (Gerber)	4½ oz.	105	26.2
Butterscotch, pudding, Junior (Gerber)	7½ oz.	195	30.7
Strained (Gerber)	4½ oz.	129	23.3
Caramel, pudding, Strained (Beech-Nut)	4¾ oz.	131	29.7
Junior (Beech-Nut)	7¾ oz.	215	48.8
Carrot, Junior (Beech-Nut)	7½ oz.	81	17.6
Junior (Gerber)	7½ oz.	63	14.9
Junior (Heinz)	7¾ oz.	86	19.0
Strained (Beech-Nut)	4½ oz.	47	10.4
Strained (Gerber)	4½ oz.	37	9.0
Strained (Heinz)	4½ oz.	52	11.6
& pea, Junior (Gerber)	7½ oz.	79	16.1
In butter sauce, Junior (Beech-Nut)	7½ oz.	119	24.2
Strained (Beech-Nut)	4½ oz.	72	15.0
Cereal, dry, barley			

Food and Description	Measure or Quantity	Calories	Carbo-hydrates (grams)
(Gerber)	3 tbsp. (7 grams)	27	5.3
Instant (Heinz)	2 tbsp.	19	3.9
High Protein (Gerber)	3 tbsp. (7 grams)	26	3.3
Hi-protein (Beech-Nut)	1 oz.	104	13.0
Instant (Heinz)	2 tbsp.	29	3.7
Mixed (Beech-Nut)	1 oz.	106	19.6
(Gerber)	3 tbsp. (7 grams)	27	5.3
(Heinz)	2 tbsp.	21	4.0
Honey (Beech-Nut)	1 oz.	106	20.0
With banana (Gerber)	3 tbsp.	28	5.5
Oatmeal (Beech-Nut)	1 oz.	108	18.8
(Gerber)	3 tbsp. (7 grams)	28	4.7
Instant (Heinz)	2 tbsp.	18	3.2
Honey (Beech-Nut)	1 oz.	109	19.8
With banana (Gerber)	3 tbsp. (7 grams)	28	5.2
Rice (Beech-Nut)	1 oz.	107	21.7
(Gerber)	3 tbsp. (7 grams)	26	5.5
Instant (Heinz)	2 tbsp.	20	4.2
Honey (Beech-Nut)	1 oz.	106	22.5
With strawberry (Gerber)	3 tbsp. (7 grams)	28	5.7
Cereal, or mixed cereal, With applesauce & banana,			
Junior (Gerber)	7-8/10 oz.	178	40.6
Strained (Gerber)	4-7/10 oz.	111	24.4
Strained (Heinz)	4¾ oz.	108	26.9
With egg yolks & bacon,			
Junior (Beech-Nut)	7½ oz.	201	17.4
Junior (Gerber)	7½ oz.	158	15.1
Junior (Heinz)	7½ oz.	164	15.5
With fruit, Strained (Beech-Nut)	4¾ oz.	113	26.0

Food and Description	Measure or Quantity	Calories	Carbohydrates (grams)
High protein with apple & banana, Strained *(Heinz)*	4¾ oz.	132	25.8
Oatmeal, with applesauce & banana, Junior *(Gerber)*	7-8/10 oz.	167	35.4
Strained *(Gerber)*	4-7/10 oz.	90	20.7
With fruit, Strained *(Beech-Nut)*	4¾ oz.	99	20.6
Rice, with applesauce & banana, Strained *(Gerber)*	4-7/10 oz.	93	21.3
Cheese, Cottage, creamed with pineapple, Junior *(Beech-Nut)*	7¾ oz.	186	35.7
Strained *(Gerber)*	4-7/10 oz.	174	23.3
With pineapple juice, Strained *(Beech-Nut)*	4¾ oz.	119	23.3
Dessert, with pineapple, Junior *(Gerber)*	7-8/10 oz.	199	37.4
Strained *(Gerber)*	4½ oz.	116	21.7
With banana, Junior *(Heinz)*	7¾ oz.	169	36.3
Strained *(Heinz)*	4½ oz.	97	20.9
Cherry vanilla, Pudding, Junior *(Gerber)*	7-8/10 oz.	190	43.3
Strained *(Gerber)*	4-7/10 oz.	115	29.8
Chicken, Junior *(Beech-Nut)*	3½ oz.	97	0
Junior *(Gerber)*	3½ oz.	133	.5
Strained *(Beech-Nut)*	3½ oz.	97	.4
Strained *(Gerber)*	3½ oz.	131	.1
& chicken broth, Junior *(Heinz)*	3½ oz.	103	0
Strained *(Heinz)*	3½ oz.	114	0
Dinner, Junior *(Beech-Nut)*	4½ oz.	105	9.0
Strained *(Beech-Nut)*	4½ oz.	110	9.3
Noodle dinner, Junior *(Beech-Nut)*	7½ oz.	95	15.5

Food and Description	Measure or Quantity	Calories	Carbohydrates (grams)
Junior *(Gerber)*	7½ oz.	93	17.0
Junior *(Heinz)*	7½ oz.	123	15.7
Strained *(Beech-Nut)*	4½ oz.	58	9.7
Strained *(Gerber)*	4½ oz.	60	10.4
Strained *(Heinz)*	4½ oz.	70	9.2
Dinner, With vegetables,			
Junior *(Beech-Nut)*	7½ oz.	98	17.6
Junior *(Gerber)*	4½ oz.	113	7.9
Junior *(Heinz)*	4¾ oz.	128	5.3
Strained *(Beech-Nut)*	4½ oz.	61	10.5
Strained *(Gerber)*	4½ oz.	110	7.7
Strained *(Heinz)*	4¾ oz.	124	5.8
Soup, Junior *(Heinz)*	7½ oz.	113	17.6
Strained *(Heinz)*	4½ oz.	65	8.9
Cream of, Junior			
(Gerber)	7½ oz.	116	19.6
Strained *(Gerber)*	4½ oz.	73	12.4
Stew, Toddler *(Gerber)*	6 oz.	128	15.0
Sticks, Junior			
(Beech-Nut)	2½ oz.	146	1.6
Junior *(Gerber)*	2½ oz.	134	.8
Cookie, Animal-shaped,			
(Gerber)	1 cookie (6 grams)	29	4.3
Assorted *(Beech-Nut)*	½ oz.	61	9.5
Corn, Creamed, Junior			
(Gerber)	7½ oz.	133	29.4
Junior *(Heinz)*	7½ oz.	153	34.0
Strained *(Beech-Nut)*	4½ oz.	123	26.5
Strained *(Gerber)*	4½ oz.	82	18.1
Strained *(Heinz)*	4½ oz.	92	20.4
Custard, Junior *(Beech-Nut)*	7¾ oz.	210	40.5
Junior *(Heinz)*	7¾ oz.	213	36.4
Strained *(Beech-Nut)*	4½ oz.	125	24.7
Strained *(Heinz)*	4½ oz.	122	21.6
Chocolate, Junior *(Gerber)*	7-8/10 oz.	208	41.1
Strained *(Beech-Nut)*	4½ oz.	138	27.8
Strained *(Gerber)*	4½ oz.	122	24.4
Vanilla, Junior *(Gerber)*	7½ oz.	202	39.7

Food and Description	Measure or Quantity	Calories	Carbohydrates (grams)
Strained *(Gerber)*	4½ oz.	112	23.4
Egg yolk, Strained			
(Beech-Nut)	3⅓ oz.	181	1.3
Strained *(Gerber)*	3-3/10 oz.	187	0
Strained *(Heinz)*	3¼ oz.	189	2.0
& bacon, Strained			
(Beech-Nut)	3⅓ oz.	174	3.3
& ham, Strained *(Gerber)*	3-3/10 oz.	182	0
Fruit, Mixed, & honey,			
Junior *(Heinz)*	7½ oz.	215	52.0
With tapioca,			
Strained *(Heinz)*	4½ oz.	105	24.7
Dessert, Junior *(Heinz)*	7¾ oz.	207	50.9
Strained *(Heinz)*	4½ oz.	124	30.4
Tropical, Junior			
(Beech-Nut)	7¾ oz.	208	51.0
With tapioca, Junior			
(Beech-Nut)	7¾ oz.	221	53.2
Junior *(Gerber)*	7-8/10 oz.	202	49.7
Strained *(Beech-Nut)*	4¾ oz.	139	34.4
Strained *(Gerber)*	4-7/10 oz.	120	29.0
Juice, Mixed, Strained			
(Beech-Nut)	4-1/5 fl. oz. (4.4 oz.)	79	19.0
Strained *(Gerber)*	4-1/5 fl. oz. (4.6 oz.)	77	18.3
Ham, Junior *(Gerber)*	3½ oz.	116	.6
Strained *(Beech-Nut)*	3½ oz.	115	2.3
Strained *(Gerber)*	3½ oz.	113	.7
Dinner, Junior			
(Beech-Nut)	4½ oz.	122	6.4
Strained *(Beech-Nut)*	4½ oz.	137	7.8
With vegetables,			
Junior *(Gerber)*	4½ oz.	100	8.3
Junior *(Heinz)*	4¾ oz.	148	12.5
Strained *(Gerber)*	4½ oz.	101	8.5
Strained *(Heinz)*	4¾ oz.	124	6.7
Lamb, Junior *(Beech-Nut)*	3½ oz.	98	0
Junior *(Gerber)*	3½ oz.	96	0

Food and Description	Measure or Quantity	Calories	Carbohydrates (grams)
Strained *(Beech-Nut)*	3½ oz.	92	0
Strained *(Gerber)*	3½ oz.	96	0
& noodles, Junior *(Beech-Nut)*	7½ oz.	151	18.2
& lamb broth, Junior *(Heinz)*	3½ oz.	97	0
Strained *(Heinz)*	3½ oz.	86	0
Liver, with liver broth, Strained *(Heinz)*	3½ oz.	79	0
Macaroni, Alphabets & beef casserole, Toddler *(Gerber)*	6-1/5 oz.	146	18.6
& bacon, Junior *(Beech-Nut)*	7½ oz.	197	20.0
& beef with vegetables, Junior *(Beech-Nut)*	7½ oz.	136	15.5
With tomato, beef & bacon, Junior *(Gerber)*	7½ oz.	132	21.9
Junior *(Heinz)*	7½ oz.	140	20.6
Strained *(Gerber)*	4½ oz.	78	11.9
Strained *(Heinz)*	4½ oz.	89	11.6
Dinner, Strained *(Beech-Nut)*	4½ oz.	108	11.0
Meat sticks, Junior *(Beech-Nut)*	2½ oz.	135	.9
Junior *(Gerber)*	2½ oz.	115	1.0
Noodles & beef, Junior *(Heinz)*	7½ oz.	111	16.4
Orange juice, Strained *(Beech-Nut)*	4-1/5 fl. oz. (4.4 oz.)	64	14.5
Strained *(Gerber)*	4-1/5 fl. oz. (4.6 oz.)	65	14.5
Strained *(Heinz)*	4½ fl. oz.	69	16.2
Orange-Apple juice, Strained *(Beech-Nut)*	4-1/5 fl. oz. (4.4 oz.)	98	23.2
Strained *(Gerber)*	4-1/5 fl. oz. (4.6 fl. oz.)	71	16.3

23

Food and Description	Measure or Quantity	Calories	Carbohydrates (grams)
Orange-apple-banana juice, Strained *(Gerber)*	4-1/5 fl. oz. (4.6 oz.)	86	20.2
Strained *(Heinz)*	4½ fl. oz.	89	21.8
Orange-apricot juice, Strained *(Beech-Nut)*	4-1/5 fl. oz. (4.4 oz.)	117	27.4
Strained *(Gerber)*	4-1/5 fl. oz. (4.6 oz.)	79	19.8
Strained *(Heinz)*	4½ fl. oz.	73	17.5
Orange-banana juice, Strained *(Beech-Nut)*	4-1/5 fl. oz.	122	28.4
Orange-pineapple juice, Strained *(Beech-Nut)*	4-1/5 fl. oz. (4.4 oz.)	104	24.7
Strained *(Gerber)*	4-1/5 fl. oz. (4.6 oz.)	78	18.6
Strained *(Heinz)*	4½ fl. oz.	72	17.5
Orange-pineapple dessert, Strained *(Beech-Nut)*	4¾ oz.	161	38.5
Orange pudding, Strained *(Heinz)*	4½ oz.	119	28.0
Strained *(Gerber)*	4-7/10 oz.	133	29.4
Pea, Strained *(Beech-Nut)*	4½ oz.	86	15.2
Strained *(Gerber)*	4½ oz.	56	10.1
Creamed, Junior *(Heinz)*	7¾ oz.	158	24.9
Strained *(Heinz)*	4½ oz.	82	12.8
In butter sauce, Junior *(Beech-Nut)*	7¼ oz.	152	25.2
Strained *(Beech-Nut)*	4½ oz.	105	17.0
Peach, Junior *(Beech-Nut)*	7¾ oz.	197	46.9
Junior *(Gerber)*	7-8/10 oz.	181	44.4
Junior *(Heinz)*	7½ oz.	247	60.1
Strained *(Beech-Nut)*	4¾ oz.	119	28.3
Strained *(Gerber)*	4-7/10 oz.	107	26.9
Strained *(Heinz)*	4½ oz.	160	37.9
Cobbler, Junior *(Gerber)*	7-8/10 oz.	192	47.1
Strained *(Gerber)*	4-7/10 oz.	116	28.5
& honey, Junior *(Heinz)*	7½ oz.	155	37.0

Food and Description	Measure or Quantity	Calories	Carbo-hydrates (grams)
With tapioca, Strained *(Heinz)*	4½ oz.	94	22.1
Melba, Junior *(Beech-Nut)*	7¾ oz.	247	59.3
Strained *(Beech-Nut)*	4¾ oz.	153	36.7
Pie. Junior *(Heinz)*	7¾ oz.	212	46.9
Strained *(Heinz)*	4¾ oz.	128	28.1
Pear, Junior *(Beech-Nut)*	7½ oz.	157	38.4
Junior *(Gerber)*	7-8/10 oz.	152	39.4
Junior *(Heinz)*	7¾ oz.	167	40.0
Strained *(Beech-Nut)*	4½ oz.	96	23.0
Strained *(Gerber)*	4-7/10 oz.	92	24.3
Strained *(Heinz)*	4½ oz.	98	23.2
& pineapple, Junior *(Beech-Nut)*	7½ oz.	167	40.7
Junior *(Gerber)*	7-8/10 oz.	156	39.5
Junior *(Heinz)*	7¾ oz.	158	38.0
Strained *(Beech-Nut)*	4½ oz.	100	24.3
Strained *(Gerber)*	4-7/10 oz.	95	24.6
Strained *(Heinz)*	4¾ oz.	104	24.9
Pineapple, Dessert, Strained *(Beech-Nut)*	4¾ oz.	142	34.7
Pineapple-orange dessert, Junior *(Heinz)*	7¾ oz.	204	49.3
Strained *(Heinz)*	4½ oz.	115	27.7
Juice Strained *(Heinz)*	4½ fl. oz.	72	16.6
Pineapple-grapefruit juice drink, Strained *(Gerber)*	4-1/5 fl. oz. (4.6 oz.)	76	18.6
Pie, Junior *(Heinz)*	7¾ oz.	237	49.5
Strained *(Heinz)*	4¾ oz.	145	30.8
Plum, with tapioca, Junior *(Beech-Nut)*	7¾ oz.	217	53.0
Junior *(Gerber)*	7-8/10 oz.	218	53.8
Strained *(Beech-Nut)*	4¾ oz.	141	34.4
Strained *(Gerber)*	4-7/10 oz.	132	32.7
Strained *(Heinz)*	4½ oz.	129	31.7
Pork, Junior *(Beech-Nut)*	3½ oz.	110	1.1
Junior *(Gerber)*	3½ oz.	113	0
Strained *(Beech-Nut)*	3½ oz.	111	.4

Food and Description	Measure or Quantity	Calories	Carbohydrates (grams)
Strained (Gerber)	3½ oz.	109	0
With pork broth, Strained (Heinz)	3½ oz.	93	0
Potatoes, Creamed, with ham, Toddler (Gerber)	6 oz.	181	18.4
Pretzel, (Gerber)	1 piece (5 grams)	19	3.9
Prune, With tapioca, Junior (Beech-Nut)	7¾ oz.	204	49.3
Junior (Gerber)	7-8/10 oz.	201	49.4
Strained (Beech-Nut)	4¾ oz.	129	31.1
Strained (Gerber)	4-7/10 oz.	118	29.3
Strained (Heinz)	4¾ oz.	140	33.7
Prune-orange juice, Strained (Beech-Nut)	4-1/5 fl. oz. (4.4 oz.)	95	22.8
Strained (Gerber)	4-1/5 fl. oz. (4.6 oz.)	99	23.6
Strained (Heinz)	4½ fl. oz.	82	19.9
Raspberry, Cobbler, Junior (Gerber)	7-8/10 oz.	180	44.4
Strained (Gerber)	4½ oz.	102	25.2
Spaghetti, & meat balls, Toddler (Gerber)	6-1/5 oz.	135	21.5
With tomato sauce & beef, Junior (Beech-Nut)	7½ oz.	159	20.1
Junior (Gerber)	7½ oz.	145	27.2
Junior (Heinz)	7½ oz.	168	26.8
With tomato sauce & meat, Strained (Heinz)	4½ oz.	96	14.6
Spinach, Creamed, Junior (Gerber)	7½ oz.	95	14.1
Strained (Gerber)	4½ oz.	53	8.3
Strained (Heinz)	4½ oz.	56	8.3
Split pea, With bacon, Junior (Gerber)	7½ oz.	179	26.6
With vegetables & bacon Junior (Heinz)	7½ oz.	213	26.6
Strained (Heinz)	4½ oz.	120	13.4

Food and Description	Measure or Quantity	Calories	Carbohydrates (grams)
& ham, Junior *(Beech-Nut)*	7½ oz.	144	23.1
Squash, Junior *(Beech-Nut)*	7½ oz.	76	16.3
Junior *(Gerber)*	7½ oz.	56	13.4
Strained *(Beech-Nut)*	4½ oz.	46	9.7
Strained *(Gerber)*	4½ oz.	35	8.2
Strained *(Heinz)*	4½ oz.	50	10.5
In butter sauce, Junior *(Beech-Nut)*	7½ oz.	108	21.4
Strained *(Beech-Nut)*	4½ oz.	64	12.7
Sweet potato, Junior *(Beech-Nut)*	7¾ oz.	136	31.3
Junior *(Gerber)*	7-8/10 oz.	153	35.9
Strained *(Beech-Nut)*	4½ oz.	73	16.9
Strained *(Gerber)*	4-7/10 oz.	92	21.7
Strained *(Heinz)*	4½ oz.	84	18.8
In butter sauce, Junior *(Beech-Nut)*	7¾ oz.	155	33.3
Strained *(Beech-Nut)*	4½ oz.	91	19.5
Teething biscuit, *(Gerber)*	1 piece (.4 oz.)	43	8.2
Tuna, With noodles, Strained *(Heinz)*	4½ oz.	55	9.3
Turkey, Junior *(Beech-Nut)*	3½ oz.	100	.7
Junior *(Gerber)*	3½ oz.	105	.1
Strained *(Beech-Nut)*	3½ oz.	104	1.0
Strained *(Gerber)*	3½ oz.	129	.3
Dinner, Junior *(Beech-Nut)*	4½ oz.	88	8.4
Strained *(Beech-Nut)*	4½ oz.	106	10.8
With rice, Junior *(Gerber)*	7½ oz.	92	15.9
Strained *(Beech-Nut)*	4½ oz.	64	12.7
Strained *(Gerber)*	4½ oz.	59	9.7
& vegetables, Junior *(Beech-Nut)*	7½ oz.	87	17.0
With vegetables, Junior *(Gerber)*	4½ oz.	101	8.3
Strained *(Gerber)*	4½ oz.	96	7.8
Strained *(Heinz)*	4¾ oz.	94	7.9

Food and Description	Measure or Quantity	Calories	Carbohydrates (grams)
Tutti-frutti dessert,			
Junior *(Heinz)*	7-¾ oz.	187	44.6
Strained *(Heinz)*	4½ oz.	108	25.1
Veal, Junior *(Beech-Nut)*	3½ oz.	88	0
Junior *(Gerber)*	3½ oz.	99	0
Strained *(Beech-Nut)*	3½ oz.	109	0
Strained *(Gerber)*	3½ oz.	89	0
Dinner, Junior *(Beech--Nut)*	4½ oz.	131	6.9
Strained *(Beech-Nut)*	4½ oz.	120	7.7
With vegetables, Junior *(Gerber)*	4½ oz.	83	9.4
Junior *(Heinz)*	4¾ oz.	109	7.1
Strained *(Gerber)*	4½ oz.	82	8.6
Strained *(Heinz)*	4¾ oz.	84	6.3
& veal broth, Junior *(Heinz)*	3½ oz.	93	0
Strained *(Heinz)*	3½ oz.	90	0
Vegetables, Garden, Strained *(Beech-Nut)*	4½ oz.	59	11.3
Strained *(Gerber)*	4½ oz.	41	7.9
Mixed, Junior *(Gerber)*	7½ oz.	85	18.4
Junior *(Heinz)*	7½ oz.	100	20.8
Strained *(Gerber)*	4½ oz.	49	10.9
& bacon, Junior *(Beech-Nut)*	7½ oz.	157	18.0
Junior *(Gerber)*	7½ oz.	137	18.7
Junior *(Heinz)*	7½ oz.	153	16.3
Strained *(Beech-Nut)*	4½ oz.	92	9.7
Strained *(Gerber)*	4½ oz.	94	13.0
Strained *(Heinz)*	4½ oz.	65	9.0
& beef, Junior *(Beech-Nut)*	7½ oz.	136	15.5
Junior *(Gerber)*	7½ oz.	108	14.7
Junior *(Heinz)*	7½ oz.	106	17.1
Strained *(Beech-Nut)*	4½ oz.	88	10.2
Strained *(Gerber)*	4½ oz.	67	8.6
Strained *(Heinz)*	4½ oz.	70	8.5
& chicken, Junior *(Gerber)*	7½ oz.	105	21.2
Strained *(Gerber)*	4½ oz.	53	9.0

Food and Description	Measure or Quantity	Calories	Carbohydrates (grams)
Dumplings, beef & bacon,			
Junior *(Heinz)*	7½ oz.	145	16.9
Strained *(Heinz)*	4½ oz.	79	10.3
Egg noodles & chicken,			
Junior *(Heinz)*	7½ oz.	134	17.6
Strained *(Heinz)*	4½ oz.	80	11.2
& turkey, Junior *(Heinz)*	7½ oz.	132	15.4
& ham, Junior *(Heinz)*	7½ oz.	132	15.4
Strained *(Beech-Nut)*	4½ oz.	82	10.5
With bacon, Junior			
(Gerber)	7½ oz.	122	18.5
Strained *(Gerber)*	4½ oz.	70	9.8
Strained *(Heinz)*	4½ oz.	79	7.3
& lamb, Junior			
(Beech-Nut)	7½ oz.	125	15.5
Junior *(Gerber)*	7½ oz.	106	16.2
Junior *(Heinz)*	7½ oz.	117	17.4
Strained *(Gerber)*	4½ oz.	64	9.9
Strained *((Heinz)*	7½ oz.	56	8.1
& liver, Junior			
(Beech-Nut)	7½ oz.	98	16.7
Strained *(Beech-Nut)*	4½ oz.	56	10.0
With bacon, Junior			
(Gerber)	7½ oz.	104	17.9
Strained *(Gerber)*	4½ oz.	77	8.4
& turkey, Junior *(Gerber)*	7½ oz.	89	17.7
Strained *(Gerber)*	4½ oz.	57	11.0
Toddler, casserole			
(Gerber)	6-1/5 oz.	158	18.0
Vegetable soup, Junior			
(Beech-Nut)	7½ oz.	85	18.2
Junior *(Heinz)*	7½ oz.	106	20.4
Strained *(Beech-Nut)*	4½ oz.	51	11.3
Strained *(Heinz)*	4½ oz.	55	10.2
BEVERAGES — NON ALCOHOLIC			
Apple Cider, *(USDA)*	½ cup	58	14.8
Cherry or sweet *(Mott's)*	½ cup	59	14.6
And cranberry juice, sweetened			
(Ocean Spray)	6 fl. oz.	110	28

Food and Description	Measure or Quantity	Calories	Carbohydrates (grams)
Apple drink, Canned *(Del Monte)*	6 fl. oz.	84	23.6
Apple Fruit drink, Canned, *(Hi-C)*	6 fl. oz.	87	22.2
Apple juice, Bottled or canned,			
(USDA)	1 cup	120	30
(Mott's)	½ cup	59	14.6
(Musselman's)	½ cup	62	
Frozen (Seneca)	½ cup (4.4 oz.)	61	14.8
(White House)	6 fl. oz.	87	22
Apple nectar *(Mott's)*	½ cup	63	15.9
Apricot-apple juice, & prune,			
(Sunsweet)	½ cup	63	16.0
Apricot-apple juice drink, Canned			
(BC)	6 fl. oz.	96	
Apricot nectar, Canned, sweetened			
(USDA)	½ cup	68	17.5
Unsweetened *(USDA)*	1 cup	140	37
Sweetened *(Del Monte)*	½ cup	68	18.0
Unsweetened *(Del Monte)*	6 fl. oz.	100	26
Sweetened *(Heinz)*	5½-fl.-oz. can	80	21.0
Sweetened *(Sunsweet)*	½ cup	75	18.0
Low calorie *(S&W Nutradiet)*	4 oz. (by. wt.)	35	8.2
(S&W Nutradiet)	6 oz.	33	9
Apricot & pineapple nectar,			
Unsweetened *(S&W Nutradiet)*	4 oz. (by. wt.)	35	8.5
(S&W Nutradiet)	6 oz.	49	12
Banana soft drink, Sweetened			
(Yoo-Hoo)	6 fl. oz.	90	18.0
High-protein *(Yoo-Hoo)*	6 fl. oz.	114	24.6
Beefamato cocktail *(Mott's)*	½ cup	49	10.7
Birch beer, Soft drink *(Pennsylvania Dutch)*	6 fl. oz.	84	19.7
(Yukon Club)	6 fl. oz.	89	22.3
Bitters *(Angostura)*	1 fl. oz.	86	12.5
Bitter lemon *(Schweppes)*	6 fl. oz.	86	12.5

* Prepared as package directs.

Food and Description	Measure or Quantity	Cal- ories	Carbo- hydrates (grams)
Bitter orange (Schweppes)	6 fl. oz.	92	22.6
Cherry fruit drink (Hi-C)	6 fl. oz.	90	
Cherry soft drink Sweetened			
(Canada Dry)	6 fl. oz.	96	24.0
(Clicquot Club)	6 fl. oz.	94	23.0
(Cott)	6 fl. oz.	94	23.0
(Fanta)	6 fl. oz.	85	21.9
(White Rock)	6 fl. oz.	89	
Cherri-Berri (Hoffman)	6 fl. oz.	91	22.8
Black (Shasta)	6 fl. oz.	88	22.2
Unsweetened or low calorie			
(Clicquot Club)	6 fl. oz.	2	.3
(Cott)	6 fl. oz.	2	.3
Black cherry (Hoffman)	6 fl. oz.	2	.4
(No-Cal)	6 fl. oz.	2	0
(Shasta)	6 fl. oz.	<1	.1
(Yukon Club)	6 fl. oz.	2	.4
Club soda soft drink, any brand, regular or dietetic.	6 fl. oz.	0	0
Carbonated water, Sweetened, Non-alcoholic (USDA)	12 fl. oz.	115	29
Coffee soft drink, Sweetened			
(Hoffman)	6 fl. oz.	70	17.5
Low calorie (Hoffman)	6 fl. oz.	3	.8
Low calorie (No-Cal)	6 fl. oz.	3	<.1
Coffee, Regular *(Chase & Sanborn)	¾ cup	1	Trace
*(Max Pax)	¾ cup	2	.5
*(Maxwell House)	¾ cup	2	.4
*(Yuban)	¾ cup	2	.4
Instant			
*(Chase & Sanborn)	¾ cup	1	Trace
Kava (Borden)	1 tsp.	3	.5
(Nescafé)	1 slightly- rounded tsp.	4	.9
(Borden)	1 rounded tsp.	5	.9

* Prepared as package directs.

Food and Description	Measure or Quantity	Calories	Carbohydrates (grams)
Dry *(USDA)	1 rounded tsp.	3	.9
Decaffeinated, Regular			
*(Sanka regular)	¾ cup	2	.4
*(Siesta)	¾ cup	1	Trace
(Decaf)	1 tsp.	4	.6
(Sanka Instant)	¾ cup	4	.9
Freeze-dried (Maxim)	¾ cup	4	.9
*(Sanka)	¾ cup	4	.8
(Tasters Choice)	1 slightly-rounded tsp.	4	.7
Cola soft drink, Sweetened			
(USDA)	12 fl. oz.	145	37
(Clicquot Club)	6 fl. oz.	83	20.0
(Coca-Cola)	6 fl. oz.	73	18.5
(Cott)	6 fl. oz.	83	20.0
(Pepsi-cola)	6 fl. oz.	78	19.5
(Royal Crown)	6 fl. oz.	81	20.4
(Shasta)	6 fl. oz.	76	19.4
(White Rock)	6 fl. oz.	80	
(Yukon Club)	6 fl. oz.	81	20.3
Cherry (Shasta)	6 fl. oz.	76	19.4
Low calorie (Canada Dry)	6 fl. oz.	<1	.1
(Clicquot Club)	6 fl. oz.	2	.1
(Cott)	6 fl. oz.	2	.1
(Diet Pepsi-Cola)	6 fl. oz.	35	8.8
(Diet Rite)	6 fl. oz.	<1	Trace
(No-Cal)	6 fl. oz.	<1	<.1
(Shasta)	6 fl. oz.	<1	<.1
(Tab)	6 fl. oz.	<1	<.1
Cherry (Shasta)	6 fl. oz.	<1	<.1
Cranberries, Cranberry juice cocktail, canned (USDA)	1 cup	165	42
(Ocean Spray)	6 fl. oz.	110	28
Low calorie (Ocean Spray)	6 fl. oz.	35	9
Cranapple, Cranberry-apple drink (Ocean Spray)	6 fl. oz.	140	34

*Prepared as package directs.

Food and Description	Measure or Quantity	Calories	Carbo-hydrates (grams)
Low calorie (Ocean Spray)	6 fl. oz.	30	7
Crangrape, Cranberry-grape drink (Ocean Spray)	6 fl. oz.	120	31
Cranicot, Cranberry-apricot drink (Ocean Spray)	6 fl. oz.	130	33
Cranprune, Cranberry-prune drink (Ocean Spray)	6 fl. oz.	130	33
Cream or Creme soft drink,			
Sweetened, Vanilla (Canada Dry)	6 fl. oz.	97	24.1
Sweetened (Clicquot Club)	6 fl. oz.	88	22.0
(Cott)	6 fl. oz.	88	22.0
(Dr. Brown's)	6 fl. oz.	84	20.9
(Fanta)	6 fl. oz.	94	24.2
(Hoffman)	6 fl. oz.	85	21.3
(Kirsch)	6 fl. oz.	77	19.6
(Nedick's)	6 fl. oz.	84	20.9
(Shasta)	6 fl. oz.	84	21.3
(Yukon Club)	6 fl. oz.	85	21.3
Low calorie (Clicquot Club)	6 fl. oz.	3	.5
(Cott)	6 fl. oz.	3	.5
(Dr. Brown's)	6 fl. oz.	1	.2
(Hoffman)	6 fl. oz.	1	.2
(No-Cal)	6 fl. oz.	2	<.1
(Shasta)	6 fl. oz.	<1	<.1
(Yukon Club)	6 fl. oz.	1	.2
Dr. Pepper soft drink,			
Regular,	6 fl. oz.	71	17.4
Sugar free,	6 fl. oz.	2	.4
Egg Nog, Dairy, 4.69% fat (Borden)	½ cup	132	16.3
8% fat (Borden)	½ cup	171	16.3
6% fat (Meadow Gold)	½ cup	164	25.5
6% butterfat (Sealtest)	½ cup	174	18.0
8% butterfat (Sealtest)	½ cup	192	17.3
With alcohol, 30 proof			
(Old Mr. Boston)	1 fl. oz.	83	4.5
Fresca soft drink	6 fl. oz.	<1	<.1
Gatorade soft drink	6 fl. oz.	53	16.0
Ginger Ale, Carbonated, Sweetened,			
(USDA)	12 fl. oz.	115	29

Food and Description	Measure or Quantity	Calories	Carbo-hydrates (grams)
(Canada Dry)	6 fl. oz.	62	16.2
(Clicquot Club)	6 fl. oz.	62	15.0
(Cott)	6 fl. oz.	62	15.0
(Fanta)	6 fl. oz.	62	15.9
(Schweppes)	6 fl. oz.	66	16.3
(Shasta)	6 fl. oz.	65	16.5
(White Rock)	6 fl. oz.	62	
Golden (Yukon Club)	6 fl. oz.	64	16.1
Pale Dry (Hoffman)	6 fl. oz.	58	14.6
(Yukon Club)	6 fl. oz.	62	15.6
Low calorie (Canada Dry)	6 fl. oz.	2	<1.0
(Clicquot Club)	6 fl. oz.	2	.5
(Cott)	6 fl. oz.	2	.5
(No-Cal)	6 fl. oz.	2	<.1
(Shasta)	6 fl. oz.	<1	<.1
Ginger beer, soft drink, Regular (Schweppes)	6 fl. oz.	72	17.6
Grape flavor Grape drink, Instant breakfast (Tang)	4 fl. oz.	50	14
Fruit drink (Hi-C)	6 oz.	98	23
Juice drink, canned (USDA)	1 cup	135	35
Grape juice, Canned or bottled (USDA)	1 cup	165	42
Frozen, concentrate, sweetened, diluted with 3 parts water by volume (USDA)	1 cup	135	33
Frozen, sweetened (Minute Maid),	6 oz.	99	25
Grape soft drink, Sweetened (Canada Dry)	6 fl. oz.	95	23.9
(Fanta)	6 fl. oz.	92	23.9
(Nehi)	6 fl. oz.	93	22.3
(Shasta)	6 fl. oz.	88	22.2
(White Rock)	6 fl. oz.	89	
Low Calorie (No-Cal)	6 fl. oz.	2	0
(Shasta)	6 fl. oz.	<1	.1
(Yukon Club)	6 fl. oz.	<1	.2
Grapefruit juice, Fresh (USDA)	1 cup	95	23
Canned, white, unsweetened			

34

Food and Description	Measure or Quantity	Calories	Carbohydrates (grams)
(USDA)	1 cup	100	24
Unsweetened (Del Monte)	6 fl. oz.	70	17
Canned, white, Sweetened			
(USDA)	1 cup	130	32
Sweetened (Del Monte)	6 fl. oz.	80	21
Dehydrated crystals prepared			
with water (USDA)	1 cup	100	24
Frozen concentrate,			
unsweetened,			
diluted with 3 parts water, by			
volume (USDA)	1 cup	80	21
Frozen (Minute Maid)	6 oz.	75	18.3
Grapefruit soft drink, Sweetened			
(Clicquot Club)	6 fl. oz.	83	20.0
(Cott)	6 fl. oz.	83	20.0
(Fanta)	6 fl. oz.	84	21.5
(Shasta)	6 fl. oz.	81	20.5
Low calorie, Golden or pink			
(Canada Dry)	6 fl. oz.	<1	<1.0
(Clicquot Club)	6 fl. oz.	3	.7
(Cott)	6 fl. oz.	3	.7
Pink (No-Cal)	6 fl. oz.	2	0
(Shasta)	6 fl. oz.	1	.1
(Shasta)	6 fl. oz.	1	.1
*Kool-Aid, Regular (General Foods)	1 cup	98	25.0
Sugar-sweetened (General Foods)	1 cup	91	23.0
Lemonade, Concentrate, frozen,			
Diluted with 4⅓ parts water, by			
volume (USDA)	1 cup	110	28
Frozen (Minute Maid)	6 oz.	74	19.6
Lemon soft drink, Sweetened			
(Canada Dry)	6 fl. oz.	88	19.2
(Clicquot Club)	6 fl. oz.	74	18.0
(Cott)	6 fl. oz.	74	18.0
Low calorie (Canada Dry)	6 fl. oz.	1	<1.0
(Clicquot Club)	6 fl. oz.	3	.5
(Cott)	6 fl. oz.	3	.5
(No-Cal)	6 fl. oz.	2	0

* Prepared as package directs

Food and Description	Measure or Quantity	Calories	Carbohydrates (grams)
Limeade, Concentrate, frozen,			
Diluted with 4⅓ parts water, by			
volume *(USDA)*	1 cup	100	27
Frozen *(Minute Maid)*	6 oz.	75	20.1
Concentrate, sweetened,			
frozen *(USDA)*	6-fl.-oz. can	408	107.9
Diluted with 4⅓ parts water			
(USDA)	½ cup	51	13.6
(ReaLemon)	6-oz. can	414	108.0
*(Minute Maid)	½ cup	50	13.4
*(Snow Crop)	½ cup	50	13.4
Limeade Mix *(Wyler's)	6 fl. oz.	64	15.8
Orange drink, Instant breakfast			
(Tang)	4 fl. oz.	50	13
(Start)	4 fl. oz.	50	13
Frozen, breakfast beverage			
(Bird's Eye Orange Plus)	6 fl. oz.	100	25
Fruit drink *(Hi-C)*	6 oz.	98	24
Orange-apricot *(USDA)*	1 cup	125	32
Orange juice, Fresh, all varieties			
(USDA)	1 cup	110	26
Canned, unsweetened *(USDA)*	1 cup	120	28
(Del Monte)	6 fl. oz.	80	19
Sweetened *(Del Monte)*	6 fl. oz.	70	18
Dehydrated crystals, prepared			
with water *(USDA)*	1 cup	115	27
Frozen concentrate diluted with			
3 parts water, by volume *(USDA)*	1 cup	120	29
(Minute Maid)	6 oz.	90	21.4
(Snow Crop)	6 oz.	90	21.4
Imitation *(Bird's Eye Awake)*	6 fl. oz.	90	23
Orange soft drink, Sweetened,			
Sunripe *(Canada Dry)*	6 fl. oz.	94	24.6
(Clicquot Club)	6 fl. oz.	103	25.0
(Cott)	6 fl. oz.	103	25.0
(Fanta)	6 fl. oz.	92	23.8
(Nedick's)	6 fl. oz.	91	22.6

*Prepared as package directs.

Food and Description	Measure or Quantity	Cal- ories	Carbo- hydrates (grams)
Low calorie *(Canada Dry)*	6 fl. oz.	<1	<1.0
(Clicquot Club)	6 fl. oz.	2	.3
(Cott)	6 fl. oz.	2	.3
(No-Cal)	6 fl. oz.	2	0
(Shasta)	6 fl. oz.	<1	<.1
Orange & grapefruit juice, Canned			
Sweetened *(Del Monte)*	6 fl. oz.	80	20
Unsweetened *(Del Monte)*	6 fl. oz.	80	19
Frozen concentrate, diluted			
With 3 parts water, by			
volume *(USDA)*	1 cup	110	26
Orange pineapple drink, *(Hi-C)*	6 oz.	98	25
Peaches, Peach nectar *(Bird's Eye)*	6 fl. oz.	100	27
(S & W Nutradiet)	6 oz.	40	9
Pear nectar, *(Del Monte)*	6 fl. oz.	110	30
(S & W Nutradiet)	6 oz.	27	6
Pineapple juice, Canned *(USDA)*	1 cup	135	34
Vitamin C fortified 2 (Del Monte)	6 fl. oz.	100	25
Pineapple grapefruit juice drink,			
(Del Monte)	6 fl. oz.	90	24
Pineapple orange juice drink,			
(Del Monte)	6 fl. oz.	90	23
Pineapple pink grapefruit juice			
drink *(Del Monte)*	6 fl. oz.	90	24
Prune juice, Canned or bottled			
(USDA)	1 cup	200	49
Unsweetened *(Bennett's)*	8 oz.	195	50
(Del Monte)	6 fl. oz.	120	33
Quinine soft drink or Tonic			
Water, Sweetened *(Canada Dry)*	6 fl. oz.	68	17.6
(Schweppes)	6 fl. oz.	66	16.5
(Yukon Club)	6 fl. oz.	67	16.7
Low calorie *(No-Cal)*	6 fl. oz.	2	0
Root Beer soft drink, Sweetened,			
Rooti *(Canada Dry)*	6 fl. oz.	76	19.6
(Clicquot Club)	6 fl. oz.	85	21.0
(Cott)	6 fl. oz.	85	21.0
(Fanta)	6 fl. oz.	77	19.8
Draft *(Shasta)*	6 fl. oz.	84	21.3

Food and Description	Measure or Quantity	Calories	Carbohydrates (grams)
(USDA)	12 fl. oz.	150	39
(Yukon Club)	6 fl. oz.	81	20.1
Low calorie (Canada Dry)	6 fl. oz.	<1	<1.0
(Clicquot Club)	6 fl. oz.	<1	<.1
(Cott)	6 fl. oz.	<1	<.1
(No-Cal)	6 fl. oz.	<1	<.1
(Yukon Club)	6 fl. oz.	<1	<.1
Draft (Shasta)	6 fl. oz.	<1	<.1
Tangerine juice, Canned, unsweetened (USDA)	1 cup	125	30
Tea, Bag (Lipton)	1 bag	0	0
(Tender Leaf)	1 bag	1	Trace
Canned (Lipton)	12 fl. oz.	138	34.6
Instant, dry powder, slightly Sweetened *(Lipton)	1 cup	0	0
(Nestea)	1 tsp.	<1	<.1
(Tender Leaf)	1 rounded tsp.	1	Trace
Lemon flavored *(Lipton)	1 cup	3	.9
Dry powder, slightly sweetened	1 tsp.	1	.4
(USDA)	1 cup	5	.9
Tea Mix, Iced, All flavors (Nestea)	3 tsp.	58	15.1
*(Salada)	1 cup	57	13.6
*(Tender Leaf)	1 cup	57	14.2
*(Wyler's)	1 cup	56	14.0
Lemon flavored (Lipton)	1 cup	102	25.5
Low calorie *(Lipton)	1 cup	4	.7
Tiki soft drink, Sweetened (Shasta)	6 fl. oz.	84	21.3
Low calorie (Shasta)	6 fl. oz.	<1	<.1
Tomato juice, Canned (Campbell's)	6 oz.	35	7
(Contadina)	6 fl. oz.	35	8
(Del Monte)	6 fl. oz.	35	8
(Hunt-Wesson)	6 oz.	35	7.8
(Libby's)	6 fl. oz.	35	8
(S & W Nutradiet)	6 oz.	35	8
(USDA)	1 cup	45	10
"V-8" Cocktail vegetable juice (Campbell's)	6 oz.	35	7

* Prepared as package directs.

38

Food and Description	Measure or Quantity	Calories	Carbohydrates (grams)
Low sodium (Campbell's)	6 oz.	35	7
Vegetable juice cocktail (S & W Nutradiet)	6 oz.	35	0

BEVERAGES—ALCOHOLIC

Food and Description	Measure or Quantity	Calories	Carbohydrates (grams)
Beer, Canned regular (Andeker)	12 fl. oz.	165	
4.9% alcohol (Budweiser)	12 fl. oz.	156	12.3
3.9% alcohol (Budweiser)	12 fl. oz.	137	11.9
4.9% alcohol (Busch Bavarian)	12 fl. oz.	156	12.3
3.9% alcohol (Busch Bavarian)	12 fl. oz.	137	11.9
(Hamm's)	12 fl. oz.	151	13.3
4.6% alcohol (Knickerbocker)	12 fl. oz.	160	13.7
4.9% alcohol (Michelob)	12 fl. oz.	160	12.8
4.7% alcohol (Narragansett)	12 fl. oz.	155	14.4
(Pabst Blue Ribbon)	12 fl. oz.	150	
4.6% alcohol (Rheingold)	12 fl. oz.	160	13.7
(Schlitz)	12 fl. oz.	155	
4.8% alcohol (Schmidt)	12 fl. oz.	165	14.9
3.2 low gravity, 3.8% alcohol (Schmidt)	12 fl. oz.	142	13.6
Low carbohydrate (Dia-beer)	12 fl. oz.	145	4.2
(Dia-beer)	7 fl. oz.	85	2.8
4.6% alcohol (Gablinger's)	12 fl. oz.	99	.2
(Meister Brau Lite)	12 fl. oz.	96	1.4
Near, Kingsbury, 4% alcohol (Heileman)	12 fl. oz.	62	15.0
Bloody Mary mix, (Bartender's)	1 serving (.3 oz.)	26	5.7
Brandy, Flavored, apricot, 70 Proof (Hiram Walker)	1 fl. oz.	88	7.5
(Old Mr. Boston)	1 fl. oz.	100	8.0
Blackberry, 70 proof (Bols)	1 fl. oz.	100	7.4
(Leroux)	1 fl. oz.	91	8.3
Cherry, 70 proof (Garnier)	1 fl. oz.	86	7.1
Coffee, 70 proof (Old Mr. Boston)	1 fl. oz.	74	1.0
Peach, 70 proof (Leroux)	1 fl. oz.	93	8.9
Champagne, 12% alcohol, brut (Gold Seal)	3 fl. oz.	85	1.4

Food and Description	Measure or Quantity	Calories	Carbohydrates (grams)
Cordon Rouge brut (Mumm's)	3 fl. oz.	65	1.4
Dry (Taylor)	3 fl. oz.	78	2.0
Extra dry (Mumm's)	3 fl. oz.	82	5.6
Cocktails, Apricot sour, Canned, Duet, 12½% alcohol (National Distillers)	2 fl. oz.	48	1.6
(Party Tyme)	2 fl. oz.	66	5.7
Liquid mix (Party Tyme)	2 fl. oz.	58	14.0
Dry mix (Party Tyme)	½-oz. pkg. 1 serving	50	11.6
Daiquiri, Canned, 52½ proof (Hiram Walker)	3 fl. oz.	177	12.0
12½% alcohol (Party Tyme)	2 fl. oz.	65	5.4
Dry mix (Bar-Tender's)	5/8-oz. serving	70	17.2
Mai Tai, Canned, duet, 12½% Alcohol (National Distillers)	8-fl.-oz. can	288	28.8
(Party Tyme)	2 fl. oz.	65	5.7
Dry mix (Bar-Tender's)	5/8-oz. serving	69	17.0
Manhattan, 55 proof (Hiram Walker)	3 fl. oz.	147	3.0
Dry mix (Bar-Tender's)	1/5 oz. 1 serving	24	5.6
Margarita, Canned, duet, 12½% Alcohol (National Distillers)	8-fl.-oz. can	248	20.0
(Party-Tyme)	2 fl. oz.	66	5.7
Dry mix (Bar-Tender's)	1 serving (5/8 oz.)	70	17.3
Martini, Canned, gin, 67.5 Proof (Hiram Walker)	3 fl. oz.	168	.6
Duet, 21% alcohol (National Distillers)	8-fl.-oz. can	560	1.6
24% alcohol (Party Tyme)	2 fl. oz.	82	0
Liquid mix (Party Tyme)	.2 fl. oz.	12	3.2
Vodka, 60 proof (Hiram Walker)	3 fl. oz.	147	0

Food and Description	Measure or Quantity	Calories	Carbohydrates (grams)
Duet, 20% alcohol			
(National Distillers)	8-fl.-oz. can	536	1.6
21% alcohol *(Party Tyme)*	2 fl. oz.	72	0
Pina Colada, Canned, 12½%			
Alcohol *(Party Tyme)*	2 fl. oz.	63	5.1
Scotch sour, Canned, duet, 12½%			
Alcohol *(National Distillers)*	8-fl.-oz.	272	25.6
(Party Tyme)	2 fl. oz.	65	5.7
Whiskey sour, Canned			
(Hiram Walker)	3 fl. oz.	177	12.0
Mix *(Bar-Tender's)*	5/8 oz. 1 serving	70	17.2
Gin, Sloe, 60 proof			
(Hiram Walker)	1 fl. oz.	68	4.8
42 proof *(Old Mr. Boston)*	1 fl. oz.	50	2.0
70 proof *(Old Mr. Boston)*	1 fl. oz.	76	1.4
Gin, Rum, Vodka, Whiskey			
86 proof *(USDA)*	1½ fl. oz.	105	Trace
90 proof *(USDA)*	1½ fl. oz.	110	Trace
100 proof *(USDA)*	1½ fl. oz.	125	Trace
Liqueurs, Abisante, 100 proof,	1 fl. oz.	87	1.0
120 proof *(Leroux)*	1 fl. oz.	104	1.0
Anisette, red or white, 60			
proof *(Old Mr. Boston)*	1 fl. oz.	90	7.5
(Hiram Walker)	1 fl. oz.	92	10.8
Apricot, 60 proof *(Bols)*	1 fl. oz.	96	8.9
(Hiram Walker)	1 fl. oz.	82	8.2
(Leroux)	1 fl. oz.	85	8.9
Aquairt, 90 proof *(Leroux)*	1 fl. oz.	75	Trace
Banana, 56 proof *(Leroux)*	1 fl. oz.	92	11.4
B & B, 86 proof *(Julius Wile)*	1 fl. oz.	94	5.7
Benedictine, 86 proof			
(Julius Wile)	1 fl. oz.	112	10.3
Blackberry, 60 proof			
(Hiram Walker)	1 fl. oz.	100	12.8
Cherry Heering, 49 proof			
(Hiram Walker)	1 fl. oz.	80	10.0
Creme De Cacao,			

Food and Description	Measure or Quantity	Calories	Carbohydrates (grams)
Brown or White,			
54 proof (Hiram Walker)	1 fl. oz.	104	15.0
(Old Mr. Boston)	1 fl. oz.	95	7.0
Creme de Menthe, Green or			
White, 60 proof (Bols)	1 fl. oz.	122	13.0
Green, 60 proof (Leroux)	1 fl. oz.	110	15.2
White, 60 proof (Leroux)	1 fl. oz.	101	12.8
Curacao, Blue, 64 proof (Bols)	1 fl. oz.	105	10.3
60 proof (Hiram Walker)	1 fl. oz.	96	11.8
Drambué, 80 proof			
(Hiram Walker)	1 fl. oz.	110	11.0
Kirsch, 96 proof (Garnier)	1 fl. oz.	83	8.8
Kummel, 70 proof			
(Hiram Walker)	1 fl. oz.	71	3.2
(Old Mr. Boston)	1 fl. oz.	78	2.0
Rock & Rye, 60 proof (Garnier)	1 fl. oz.	70	6.2
(Hiram Walker)	1 fl. oz.	87	9.5
Irish Moss, 70 proof (Leroux)	1 fl. oz.	110	13.0
48 proof (Old Mr. Boston)	1 fl. oz.	72	6.0
60 proof (Old Mr. Boston)	1 fl. oz.	94	5.8
Israeli, Sabra (Park Avenue Imports)	1 fl. oz.	91	10.4
Tia Maria, 63 proof			
(Hiram Walker)	1 fl. oz.	92	10.0
Vermouth, Dry & extra dry, 19%			
Alcohol (C & P)	3 fl. oz.	90	3.0
18% alcohol (Gallo)	3 fl. oz.	75	1.7
18.5% alcohol (Lejon)	3 fl. oz.	99	2.2
19% alcohol (Noilly Pratt)	3 fl. oz.	101	1.6
17% alcohol (Taylor)	3 fl. oz.	102	.9
Sweet, 16% alcohol (C & P)	3 fl. oz.	120	14.4
18% alcohol (Gallo)	3 fl. oz.	118	12.3
18.5% alcohol (Lejon)	3 fl. oz.	134	11.4
16% alcohol (Noilly Pratt)	3 fl. oz.	128	12.1
17% alcohol (Taylor)	3 fl. oz.	132	10.4
White, 16.8% alcohol (Gancia)	3 fl. oz.	132	7.8
18.5% alcohol (Lejon)	3 fl. oz.	101	2.6
Wine, Bali Hai, 11% alcohol (Italian Swiss			

Food and Description	Measure or Quantity	Calories	Carbohydrates (grams)
Colony-Gold Medal)	3 fl. oz.	89	9.2
Beaujolais, French Burgundy,			
12% alcohol (Barton & Guestier)	3 fl. oz.	60	.1
(Cruse)	3 fl. oz.	72	
11% alcohol (Chanson)	3 fl. oz.	78	6.3
Beaune, St. Vincent, French			
Burgundy, 12% alcohol			
(Chanson)	3 fl. oz.	84	6.3
Clos des Feves (Chanson)	3 fl. oz.	84	6.3
Bernkasteler, German Moselle,			
11% alcohol (Deinhard)	3 fl. oz.	60	1.0
Blackberry, 12% alcohol			
(Mogen David)	3 fl. oz.	135	
Burgundy, Sparkling, 12%			
alcohol (Italian Swiss			
Colony-Private Stock)	3 fl. oz.	67	2.3
(Great Western)	3 fl. oz.	88	5.0
(Taylor)	3 fl. oz.	78	1.8
(Private Stock/Italian			
Swiss Colony)	3 fl. oz.	60	.2
American (Mogen David)	3 fl. oz.	24	1.8
12½% alcohol (Taylor)	3 fl. oz.	72	Trace
13% alcohol (Gallo)	3 fl. oz.	52	.9
Catawba, Pink, 13% alcohol			
(Great Western)	3 fl. oz.	116	11.0
13-14% alcohol (Gold Seal)	3 fl. oz.	125	9.8
Chablis, Pink, 13% alcohol			
(Gallo)	3 fl. oz.	61	3.0
12% alcohol (Great Western)	3 fl. oz.	76	1.7
12½% alcohol			
(Louis M. Martini)	3 fl. oz.	90	.2
Chianti, Classico, 12½%			
alcohol (Antinori)	3 fl. oz.	87	6.3
(Louis M. Martini)	3 fl. oz.	90	.2
Claret, 12½% alcohol			
(Louis M. Martini)	3 fl. oz.	90	.2
(Taylor)	3 fl. oz.	72	Trace
Cold Duck, 12% alcohol			
(Italian Swiss Colony-			

Food and Description	Measure or Quantity	Calories	Carbohydrates (grams)
Private Stock)	3 fl. oz.	75	4.3
Concord, 12% alcohol			
(Mogen David)	3 fl. oz.	120	16.0
Dessert (USDA)	3½ fl. oz.	140	8
Madeira, 19% alcohol (Leacock)	3 fl. oz.	120	6.3
Marsala, 19.7% alcohol			
(Italian Swiss Colony			
-Private Stock)	3 fl. oz.	124	7.1
May, 11% alcohol (Deinhard)	3 fl. oz.	60	1.0
Moselmaid, German Moselle, 1			
alcohol (Deinhard)	3 fl. oz.	60	1.0
Muscatel, 14% alcohol (Gallo)	3 fl. oz.	86	7.9
16% alcohol (Gallo)	3 fl. oz.	92	7.3
20% alcohol (Gallo)	3 fl. oz.	111	8.3
Orvieto, Italian white, 12%			
alcohol (Antinori)	3 fl. oz.	84	6.3
Paisano, 13% alcohol (Gallo)	3 fl. oz.	81	6.8
Port, 16% alcohol (Gallo)	3 fl. oz.	94	7.8
Ruby, 20% alcohol (Gallo)	3 fl. oz.	112	8.8
White, 20% alcohol (Gallo)	3 fl. oz.	111	8.3
Rosé, 11-14% alcohol			
(Château Ste. Roseline)	3 fl. oz.	84	6.3
Gypsy, 20% alcohol (Gallo)	3 fl. oz.	112	9.1
Isabella, 12% alcohol (Great			
Western)	3 fl. oz.	84	3.8
Grenache, 12.4% alcohol (Italian			
Swiss Colony-Gold Metal)	3 fl. oz.	69	2.2
Gamay, 12½% alcohol			
(Louis M. Martini)	3 fl. oz.	90	.2
12% alcohol (Mogen David)	3 fl. oz.	75	8.9
Vin Rosé d'Anjou, 12% alcohol			
(Nectarosé)	3 fl. oz.	70	2.6
12½% alcohol (Taylor)	3 fl. oz.	69	Trace
Sauternes, French white			
Bordeaux, 13% alcohol			
(Barton & Guestier)	3 fl. oz.	95	7.6
12%alcohol (Gallo)	3 fl. oz.	50	.8
Dry, 12% alcohol (Gold Seal)	3 fl. oz.	82	.4
(Mogen David)	3 fl. oz.	30	1.8

Food and Description	Measure or Quantity	Cal- ories	Carbo- hydrates (grams)
12½% alcohol (Louis M. Martini)	3 fl. oz.	90	.2
12½ alcohol (Taylor)	3 fl. oz.	81	2.9
Table (USDA)	3½ fl. oz.	85	4
Thunderbird, 14% alcohol (Gallo)	3 fl. oz.	86	8.1
20% alcohol (Gallo)	3 fl. oz.	106	7.5
BREADS			
Bagel, 3 in. diam., egg (USDA)	1 bagel	165	28
Water (USDA)	1 bagel	165	30
Biscuits, Baking powder (1869 Brand)	2 biscuits	210	26
From mix, 2 in. diam. (USDA)	1 biscuit	90	15
From home recipe with enriched flour, 2 in. diam., (USDA)	1 biscuit	105	13
Buttermilk (1869 Brand)	2 biscuits	210	26
(Pillsbury)	2 biscuits	110	21
Flaky (Hungry Jack)	2 biscuits	180	23
Oven ready (Ballard)	2 biscuits	120	22
Biscuit Dough, Refrigerated *Big 10's (Borden)	1 biscuit (1 oz.)	107	15.8
*Germ (Borden)	1 biscuit (1 oz.)	100	11.0
Biscuit Mix, Bisquick (Betty Crocker)	1 cup	503	79.4
Breads, Brown bread, plain (B & M)	1 oz.	52	11.4
Boston brown bread, slice 3 in. by ¾ in. (USDA)	1 slice	100	22
Canned bread, Brown with raisins (B & M)	½-in. slice (1.6 oz.)	78	16.5
Date & Nut (Crosse & Blackwell)	½-in.-slice (1 oz.)	65	12.6
(Dromedary)	½-in. slice (1 oz.)	74	12.8
Cinnamon raisin loaf (Thomas')	1 slice	60	12.2
Corn bread, Easy mix (Aunt Jemima's)	1/6 of corn bread	228	34.9

*Prepared as package directs.

Food and Description	Measure or Quantity	Calories	Carbohydrates (grams)
(Ballard)	1/8 recipe	160	26
French bread (Pepperidge Farm)	2 oz.	150	27
(Wonder)	2 oz.	150	28
French or Vienna, enriched 1 lb. loaf (USDA)	1 loaf	1315	251
French toast, frozen (Aunt Jemima)	2 slices	175	27.2
(Eggo)	1 slice	80	13
With link sausages, frozen breakfast (Swanson)	4½ oz.	300	22
Italian bread (Pepperidge Farm)	2 oz.	140	27
Italian bread, enriched, 1 lb. loaf (USDA)	1 loaf	1250	256
Melba thin, diet slice (Arnold)	.6 oz. slice	44	6.7
Natural health (Arnold)	.9 oz. slice	73	10.8
Oatmeal (Arnold)	.8 oz. slice	64	10.9
Pumpernickel, loaf, 1 lb. (USDA)	1 loaf	1115	241
Jewish (Arnold)	1.4-oz. slice	104	18.9
Raisin, 18 slices per loaf (USDA)	1 slice	65	13
Raisin rounds (Wonder)	2 oz.	150	28
Rye, American, light, 18 slices per loaf (USDA)	1 slice	60	13
(Wonder)	2 oz.	150	27
Melba think, Jewish (Arnold)	.6 oz. slice	43	7.8
Party (Pepperidge Farm)	1 slice (6 grams)	16	3.0
Vienna, 20 slices to 1 lb. (USDA)	.8 oz. slice	67	12.7
Wheat (Wonder)	2 oz.	150	27
Cracked wheat (Wonder)	2 slices	150	27
18 slices per loaf (USDA)	1 slice	65	13
Whole-wheat, soft-crumb type, 16 slices per loaf (USDA)	1 slice	65	14
Whole-wheat, firm-crumb type, 18 slices per loaf (USDA)	1 slice	60	12
100% Whole wheat (S.B. Thomas)	1 slice	50	10.6
White enriched, slice toasted	1 slice	70	13
Firm-crumb type, 20 slices per loaf (USDA)	1 slice	65	12
White, large (Pepperidge Farm)	2 slices	150	27
Sandwich (Pepperidge Farm)	2 slices	120	24

Food and Description	Measure or Quantity	Calories	Carbohydrates (grams)
Very thin (Pepperidge Farm)	2 slices	90	16
White, enriched (Wonder)	2 oz.	150	27
Enriched soft-crumb type, 18 slices per loaf (USDA)	1 slice	70	13
Bread crumbs, dry, grated (USDA)	1 cup	390	73
Bread dough, frozen (Morton)	1 oz.	82	15.2
Bread mix, Banana (Pillsbury)	1/16 loaf	110	20
Date (Pillsbury)	1/16 loaf	120	23
Nut (Pillsbury)	1/16 loaf	120	20
Bread stick, Cheese (Keebler)	1 pc. (3 g.)	10	1.8
Dietetic (Stella D'Oro)	1 pc. (9 g.)	39	6.3
Garlic (Keebler)	1 pc. (3 g.)	11	1.9
Onion (Keebler)	1 pc. (3 g.)	10	1.9
Regular (Stella D'Oro)	1 pc. (10g.)	40	6.6
Salt (USDA)	1 pc. (3 g.)	12	2.3
Sesame (Keebler)	1 pc. (3 g.)	11	1.8
Bread stuffing mix, cooked With butter (Uncle Ben's Stuff 'n' Such)	½ cup	191	24.3
Cooked without butter (Uncle's Ben's Stuff 'n' Such)	½ cup	118	24.2
Matzo, Regular (Manischewitz)	1 matzo (1.1 oz.)	114	28.1
American (Manischewitz)	1 matzo (1 oz.)	121	22.6
Diet-10's (Goodman's)	1 small square (1/9 of matzo)	12	2.5
(Goodman's)	1 matzo (1 oz.)	109	23.0
Diet-thins (Manischewitz)	1 matzo (1 oz.)	113	24.5
Egg (Manischewitz)	1 matzo (1.2 oz.)	133	26.6
Egg 'n Onion (Manischewitz)	1 matzo (1 oz.)	116	24.6
Onion Tams (Manischewitz)	1 piece	13	1.9

Food and Description	Measure or Quantity	Calories	Carbo-hydrates (grams)
Tam Tams *(Manischewitz)*	1 piece	14	1.7
Tasteas *(Manischewitz)*	1 matzo (1 oz.)	119	24.2
Tea *(Goodman's)*	1 matzo (.6 oz.)	70	12.9
Midgetea *(Goodman's)*	1 matzo (.4 oz.)	40	7.4
Thin tea *(Manischewitz)*	1 matzo) (1 oz.)	114	24.8
Unsalted *(Goodman's)*	1 matzo (1 oz.)	109	23.0
(Horowitz-Margareten)	1 matzo (1.2 oz.)	135	28.2
Whole wheat *(Manischewitz)*	1 matzo (1.2 oz.)	124	24.2
Matzo meal *(Manischewitz)*	1 cup (4.1 oz.)	438	96.2
Muffins, Muffin mix *(Duncan Hines)*	1 muffin	90	16
With enriched white flour, 3 in. diam. *(USDA)*	1 muffin	120	17
Blueberry, frozen *(Morton)*	1.58 oz.	120	22
Corn muffin rounds, frozen, 9 oz. *(Morton)*	1.50 oz.	130	20
10 oz. *(Morton)*	1.66 oz.	130	20
Corn muffins *(S. B. Thomas)*	1 muffin	185	25.9
Corn muffins, made with enriched degermed, cornmeal & enriched flour, 2-3/8 in. diam. *(USDA)*	1 muffin	125	19
Corn muffin mix *(Flako)*	1 medium-sized muffin	133	20.7
Corn muffins made with mix, egg & milk, 2-3/8 in. diam. *(USDA)*	1 muffin	130	20
English *(S. B. Thomas)*	1 muffin	130	26.8
(Wonder)	2 oz.	130	26
English, onion *(S. B. Thomas)*	1 muffin	135	26.8
Sour dough *(Wonder)*	2 oz.	130	27

Food and Description	Measure or Quantity	Calories	Carbohydrates (grams)
Wheat berry (Wonder)	2 oz.	130	27
Popovers, Popover mix (Flako)	1 large popover	163	22.7
Rolls, Butter crescent rolls (Pepperidge Farm)	1 roll	130	14
Cloverleaf or pan rolls, home recipe (USDA)	1 roll	120	20
Commercial (USDA)	1 roll	85	15
Dinner rolls (Pillsbury)	1 roll	100	17
Crescent rolls (Ballard)	2 rolls	190	26
Deli rolls, plain, seeded (Pepperidge Farm)	1 roll	160	30
Dinner rolls (Pepperidge Farm)	2 rolls	120	19
(Wonder)	2 oz.	170	27
Frankfurter or hamburger roll (USDA)	1 roll	120	21
French rolls, large (Pepperidge Farm)	½ roll	180	36
Hamburger (Pepperidge Farm)	1 roll	110	19
Hamburger or hot dog bun (Wonder)	2 oz.	160	29
Hard, round, or rectangular rolls (USDA)	1 roll	155	30
Hot roll mix (Pillsbury)	2 rolls	190	31
Parkerhouse rolls (Pepperidge Farm)	3 rolls	170	28
(Pillsbury)	2 rolls	120	23
Snowflake (Pillsbury)	2 rolls	140	23
Sweet rolls, cinnamon with icing (Pillsbury)	2 rolls	230	34
Stuffing mix, Chicken (Stove Top)	½ cup	180	20
Cornbread (Stove Top)	½ cup	170	20
Stuffing mix with rice (Stove Top)	½ cup	180	23
Wafers, Rye wafers, whole grain, 1-7/8 by 3½ in. (USDA)	2 wafers	45	10

CAKES

Angel Food, Home recipe (USDA)	1/12 of 8		

Food and Description	Measure or Quantity	Calories	Carbo-hydrates (grams)
	in. cake	108	24.1
Cake mix, piece 1/12 of 10 in. diam. cake (USDA)	1 piece	135	32
Made from Cake Mix (Duncan Hines)	1/12 cake	130	30
(Swansdown)	1/12 cake	132	29.7
White (Pillsbury)	1/12 cake	140	33
Raspberry swirl (Pillsbury)	1 oz.	102	23.6
Traditional angel food (Betty Crocker)	1/12 pkg.	140	32
Apple cake, mix, cinnamon pudding cake (Betty Crocker)	1/6 cake	223	44.5
Cinnamon, upside down (Betty Crocker)	1/9 cake	269	44.2
Applesauce raisin, mix (Duncan Hines)	1/9 cake	200	37
Applesauce spice layer cake, mix (Pillsbury)	1/12 cake	200	34
Boston Cream pie, piece 1/12 of 8 in. diam. (USDA)	1 piece	210	34
Mix (Betty Crocker)	1/8 pie	265	47.9
Banana cake mix, Layer *(Betty Crocker)	1/12 cake	205	36.6
(Pillsbury)	1 oz.	120	22.7
Loaf cake (Pillsbury)	1 oz.	117	22.6
Banana Supreme mix (Duncan Hines)	1/12 cake	200	35
Butter cake, white, mix (Pillsbury)	1/12 cake	190	32
Golden (Duncan Hines)	1/12 cake	280	37
Bundt Cake mix, Devil's food (Pillsbury)	1/12 cake	250	32
German chocolate (Pillsbury)	1/12 cake	250	33
Marble supreme (Pillsbury)	1/12 cake	330	50
Pound cake (Pillsbury)	1/12 cake	330	44
Yellow cake (Pillsbury)	1/12 cake	260	33
Cheese Cake, Frozen (Mrs. Smith's) 1/6 of 8 in.	cake	306	38.8

*Prepared as package directs.

Food and Description	Measure or Quantity	Calories	Carbo-hydrates (grams)
Mix *(Jello)	(4 oz.) 1/8 cake incl. crust (3.3 oz.)	255	31.4
Mis "No-Bake" *(Royal)	1/8 of 9 in. cake incl. crust (3.2 oz.)	240	28.8
Chiffon Cake mix, Lemon (Betty Crocker)	1/12 cake	190	35
Chocolate Cake, Home recipe, With chocolate icing,	1/16 of 10 in. cake	443	67.0
2 layer (USDA)	1/16 of 9 in. cake	277	41.8
With uncooked white icing (USDA)	1/16 of 10 in. cake	443	71.0
Without icing (USDA)	3 oz.	311	44.2
Chocolate Fudge mix (Pillsbury)	1/12 cake	210	34
Fudge Supreme mix (Betty Crocker)	1/12 cake	200	34
Chocolate Malt layer mix (Betty Crocker)	1/12 cake	200	35.8
Chocolate Pudding mix (Betty Crocker)	6 cake	221	44.0
Deep Chocolate mix (Duncan Hines)	1/12 cake	201	34.2
Frozen, frosted (Sara Lee)	1 oz.	102	16.0
Frozen, fudge (Pepperidge Farm)	1/6 cake	315	43.4
Fudge, Sour cream, shocolate flavor layer, mix (Betty Crocker)	1/12 cake	195	35.4
Fudge Marble cake mix (Duncan Hines)	1/12 cake	200	35
(Duncan Hines)	1/12 cake	202	35.0
Fudge, Macaroon, mix (Pillsbury)	1 oz.	124	21.2

*Prepared as package directs.

C
D

Food and Description	Measure or Quantity	Calories	Carbohydrates (grams)
Fudge, Butter recipe (Duncan Hines)	1/12 cake	283	35.2
Funny Bones, Chocolate (Drake's)	1-3/8-oz. cake	163	19.5
German Chocolate, Frozen (Morton)	2.2 oz. serving	230	28.0
(Sara Lee)	1 oz.	91	12.0
German Chocolate mix (Betty Crocker)	1/12 cake	200	34
(Pillsbury)	1 oz.	121	22.0
(Swansdown)	1/12 cake	187	35.8
Layer cake mix (Betty Crocker)	1/12 cake	200	35.9
(Pillsbury)	1/12 cake	210	35
Golden, Frozen chocolate cake (Pepperidge Farm)	1/6 cake	320	43.6
Marble Cake mix, Chocolate (Betty Crocker)	1/12 cake	200	34
Milk Chocolate layer mix (Betty Crocker)	1/12 cake	199	35.0
(Van de Kamp's)	2 layer	2825	
Swiss Chocolate mix (Duncan Hines)	1/12 cake	201	34.2
Coffee Cake, easy mix (Aunt Jemima)	1/8 cake	186	30.3
Butter pecan, mix (Pillsbury)	1/8 cake	310	39
Cinnamon streusal, mix (Pillsbury)	1/8 cake	250	41
Junior (Drake's)	1 cake	149	22.0
Large (Drake's)	11-oz. cake	1426	211.6
Small (Drake's)	1 pkg.	290	43.1
Bear Claw (Van de Kamp's)	1 piece	127	
Blueberry ring, Frozen (Sara Lee)	1 oz.	108	15.0
Butterfly (Mrs. Smith's)	1 piece	250	28.4
Cherry (Mrs. Smith's)	1 piece	240	25.5
Cinnamon-raisin (Mrs. Smith's)	1 piece	295	42.5

Food and Description	Measure or Quantity	Calories	Carbohydrates (grams)
Cinnamon Twist (*Pepperidge Farm*)	1/6 cake	156	21.3
Danish, apple, frozen (*Morton*)	1 cake	1130	166.6
(*Sara Lee*)	1 oz.	84	11.0
Danish, cherry, frozen (*Sara Lee*)	1 oz.	75	11.0
Danish Pastry, without fruit or nuts, individual round (*USDA*)	1 piece	274	29.6
Packaged ring (*USDA*)	12-oz. cake	1435	155.0
Danish pecan twist, frozen (*Morton*)	12-oz. cake	1369	149.4
Lemon ring (*Drake's*)	13-oz. cake	1028	217.3
Melt-A-Way, frozen (*Morton*)	13-oz. cake	1511	184.8
Meltaway (*Mrs. Smith's*)	1 piece	340	25.5
Pecan ring (*Drake's*)	13-oz. cake	1109	210.8
Pecan roll (*Mrs. Smith's*)	1 piece	395	48.2
Raspberry ring (*Drake's*)	13 oz.	1028	199.6
Frozen (*Sara Lee*)	1 oz.	109	15.0
Cupcakes, 2½ in. diam. without icing (*USDA*)	1 cupcake	90	14
Home recipe, with chocolate icing (*USDA*)	2¾-in. cake	184	29.7
With boiled white icing (*USDA*)	2¾-in. cake	176	30.9
With uncooked white icing (*USDA*)	¾-in. cake	184	31.6
With chocolate icing (*USDA*)	2¼-in. cake	130	21
Without icing (*USDA*)	2¾-in. cake	146	22.4
Commercial cupcakes, Devil's, food cake			
2 to pkg. (*Hostess*)	1 cake	160	29.6
12 to pkg. (*Hostess*)	1 cake	122	22.5
Orange, 2 to pkg. (*Hostess*)	1 cake	150	26.7
12 to pkg. (*Hostess*)	1 cake	133	23.7
Orange, Creme filled (*Tastykake*)	1 cake	133	17.1
Twinkies, golden sponge (*Hostess*)	2 cakes	320	52
Chocolate (*Tastykake*)	1 cake	192	33.0

Food and Description	Measure or Quantity	Calories	Carbohydrates (grams)
Creme filled *(Drake's)*	1 cake	187	25.6
Chocolate creme filled *(Tastykake)*	1 cake	128	23.2
Coconut *(Tastykake)*	1 cake	92	16.7
Creme filled, Chocolate butter cream *(Tastykake)*	1 cake	161	23.1
Golden, Creme filled *(Drake's)*	1 cake	172	21.6
Lemon, Creme filled *(Tastykake)*	1 cake	124	17.1
Raisin Snack, Junior *(Drake's)*	1 cake	112	19.2
Small *(Drake's)*	1 cake	233	41.8
Vanilla, Creme filled *(Tastykake)*	1 cake	123	16.4
Vanilla, Triplets *(Tastykake)*	1 cake	101	16.1
Cupcake mix* *(USDA)*	4 oz.	497	86.0
Without icing *(USDA)*	1 cake (.9 oz.)	88	14.0
With chocolate icing *(USDA)*	1 cake (1.2 oz.)	129	21.3
(Flako)	1 large cake	140	21.9
(Flako)	8-oz. cake	101	15.9
Devil's food *(Betty Crocker)*	1/12 cake	200	34
(Duncan Hines)	1/12 cake	200	34
2 layer cake, with chocolate icing, 1/16 of 9 in. diam. cake *(USDA)*	1 piece	235	40
Fruitcake, dark, Home recipe *(USDA)*	2 × 2 × ½ in. slice	144	17.9
(USDA)	1-lb. loaf	1719	270.8
Made with enriched flour, Slice, 1/30 of 8 in. loaf *(USDA)*	1 slice	55	9
Fruitcake, light, Home recipe *(USDA)*	2 × 2 × ½ in. slice of 1-lb loaf	117	17.2
(USDA)	1-lb. loaf	1765	260.4
Fruit 'N Crunch, Bar mix, apple			

*Prepared as package directs.

Food and Description	Measure or Quantity	Calories	Carbohydrates (grams)
(Pillsbury)	2-in. square	140	18
Bar mix, cherry (Pillsbury)	2-in. square	150	20
Gingerbread (Pillsbury)	3-in. square	190	36
1/9 of 8 in. square cake (USDA)	1 piece	175	32
Lemon cake (Pillsbury)	1/12 cake	200	33
Sunkist lemon (Betty Crocker)	1/12 cake	200	13
Lemon supreme cake (Duncan Hines)	12 cake	200	35
Orange supreme *(Duncan Hines)	1/12 cake	201	35.0
Sunkist Orange (Betty Crocker)	1/12 cake	200	34
Pound Cake, Frozen (Morton)	1 oz.	117	14.8
(Sara Lee)	1 oz.	110	13.0
Commercial (Drake's)	9-oz. cake	910	147.4
Plain (Drake's)	1 slice (1½-oz.)	171	27.8
Commercial (Drake's)	1.1-oz. slice	104	
All butter, Jr. (Drake's)	1.5-oz. slice	142	
Commercial, Raisin (Drake's)	1½-oz. slice	210	34.0
Mix (Betty Crocker)	1/12 cake	210	28.0
(Dromedary)	1-in. slice	313	40.7
Home Recipe, Traditional (USDA)	1 slice 3 × 3½ × ½-in.	123	16.4
Slice ½-in. thick (USDA)	1 slice	140	14
Plain sheet cake, with boiled white icing, piece 1/9 of 9-in. square cake (USDA)	1 piece	400	71
Pudding cake mix, Chocolate *(Betty Crocker)	1/6 pkg.	230	45
Snack cake mix, Banana nut (Duncan Hines)	1/9 cake	190	31
Double chocolate chip (Duncan Hines)	1/9 cake	180	32

*Prepared as package directs.

Food and Description	Measure or Quantity	Cal-ories	Carbo-hydrates (grams)
Snackin' cake mix, Chocolate chip (Betty Crocker)	1/9 pkg.	220	35
Spice raisin (Betty Crocker)	1/9 pkg.	200	34
Sour cream cake, White (Betty Crocker)	1/12 cake	200	34
Yellow (Betty Crocker)	1/12 cake	200	34
Spice Cake (Duncan Hines)	1/12 cake	200	35
Sponge cake, Piece 1/12 of 10--in. diam. cake (USDA)	1 piece	195	36
Streusel Swirl, Devil's food (Pillsbury)	1/12 cake	330	47
Lemon (Pillsbury)	1/12 cake	340	49
Spice (Pillsbury)	1/12 cake	350	48
Toffee Cake (Pillsbury)	1 oz.	119	21.7
White cake mix, Whipping cream (Pillsbury)	1/12 cake	177	36.2
Sour cream layer (Betty Crocker)	1/12 cake	191	34.1
(Pillsbury)	1/12 cake	200	35
(Duncan Hines)	1/12 cake	190	36
(Betty Crocker)	1/12 cake	200	35
2 layer cake with chocolate icing, 1/16 of 9 in. diam. (USDA)	1 piece	250	45
Yellow cake mix (Pillsbury)	1/12 cake	200	33
(Duncan Hines)	1/12 cake	200	35
(Betty Crocker)	1/12 cake	190	34
Butter recipe (Betty Crocker)	1/12 cake	278	37.0
Butter flavor (Pillsbury)	1 oz.	122	21.9
Yellow layer cake (Betty Crocker)	1/12 cake	202	35.5
2-layer without icing, piece 16 of 9-in. diam. cake (USDA)	1 piece	200	32
2-layer With chocolate icing, piece 1/16 of 9-in. diam. cake (USDA)	1 piece	275	45

Cake icings: See Sugar, Sweets

*Prepared as package directs.

Food and Description	Measure or Quantity	Calories	Carbohydrates (grams)
CAKE NEEDS			
Baking Chocolate, bitter or			
baking (USDA)	1 oz.	145	8
(Hershey's)	1 oz.	169	6.6
Bitter or unsweetened (Baker's)	1-oz. square	136	7.7
Grated (USDA)	½ cup	333	19.1
Pre-melted (Choco-Bake)	1-oz. packet	172	10.2
Sweetened, Bittersweet (USDA)	1 oz.	135	13.3
Milk chocolate chips			
(Hershey's)	1 oz.	152	15.9
Semi-sweet, small pieces			
(USDA)	1 cup	869	97
Chocolate chips (Baker's)	¼ cup	191	28.5
Dark flavored baking chips			
(Hershey's)	¼ cup	210	23
German's sweet (Baker's)	1 oz. (4½ in. sq.)	141	16.9
Milk Chocolate Morsels			
(Nestle's)	1 oz.	152	18.0
Morsels, Semisweet (Nestle's)	6-oz. pkg.	820	108.4
	1 oz.	137	18.1
Semisweet (Baker's)	1-oz. square	132	16.7
Baking Powder, Regular, Phosphate			
(USDA)	1 tsp. (5 grams)	6	1.4
SA8 (USDA)	1 tsp. (4 grams)	5	1.2
Tartrate (USDA)	1 tsp. (4 grams)	3	.7
(Calumet)	1 tsp. (4 grams)	2	.5
(Royal)	1 tsp. (4 grams)	5	1.3
Low sodium, commercial (USDA)	1 tsp. (4 grams)	6	1.5

Food and Description	Measure or Quantity	Calories	Carbohydrates (grams)
Yeast, Baker's dry, active			
(USDA)	1 pkg.	20	3
(Fleischmann's)	1 pkg.	20	2.9
Active, cake (Fleischmann's)	1 cake	20	1.9
Brewer's, dry (USDA)	1 tbsp.	25	3
CANDY — NONCOMMERCIAL			
Almond, Chocolate-coated (USDA)	1 oz.	161	11.2
Sugar-coated or Jordan (USDA)	1 oz.	129	19.9
Butterscotch (USDA)	1 oz.	113	26.9
Candy Corn (USDA)	1 oz.	103	25.4
Caramels, plain or chocolate			
(USDA)	1 oz.	115	22
Plain with nuts (USDA)	1 oz.	121	20.0
Chocolate flavored roll			
(USDA)	1 oz.	112	23.4
Chocolate, Semisweet (USDA)	1 oz.	144	16.2
Sweet (USDA)	1 oz.	150	16.4
Bittersweet (USDA)	1 oz.	135	13.3
Milk chocolate plain (USDA)	1 oz.	145	16
Milk chocolate with peanuts			
(USDA)	1 oz.	154	12.6
Milk chocolate with almonds			
(USDA)	1 oz.	151	14.5
Chocolate discs, sugar coated			
(USDA)	1 oz.	132	20.6
Chocolate coated peanuts			
(USDA)	1 oz.	160	11
Coconut center, Chocolate-			
-coated (USDA)	1 oz.	124	20.4
Fondant, Plain (USDA)	1 oz.	103	25.4
Chocolate-covered (USDA)	1 oz.	116	23.0
Fudge, Chocolate (USDA)	1 oz.	115	21
Chocolate-coated (USDA)	1 oz.	122	20.7
With nuts (USDA)	1 oz.	121	19.6
With nuts, Chocolate-coated			
(USDA)	1 oz.	128	19.1
Vanilla fudge (USDA)	1 oz.	113	21.2
With nuts (USDA)	1 oz.	120	19.5

Food and Description	Measure or Quantity	Calories	Carbohydrates (grams)
Fudge with peanuts & caramel, Chocolate-coated (USDA)	1 oz.	130	16.6
Gumdrops (USDA)	1 oz.	100	25
Hard Candy (USDA)	1 oz.	110	28
Honeycombed hard candy, with Peanut butter, chocolate-covered (USDA)	1 oz.	131	20.0
Jelly Beans (USDA)	1 oz.	104	26.4
Marshmallows (USDA)	1 oz.	90	23
Mints, Uncoated (USDA)	1 oz.	103	25.4
Nougat & caramel, Chocolate Covered (USDA)	1 oz.	118	20.6
Peanut bar (USDA)	1 oz.	146	13.4
Peanut Brittle (USDA)	1 oz.	119	23.0
Peanuts, Chocolate-covered (USDA)	1 oz.	159	11.1
Raisins, Chocolate-covered (USDA)	1 oz.	120	20.0
Vanilla creams, Chocolate-covered (USDA)	1 oz.	123	19.9

CANDY — COMMERCIAL

Food and Description	Measure or Quantity	Calories	Carbohydrates (grams)
Air Bon (Whitman's)	1 piece	10	
Almond, Chocolate-covered, Candy -Coated (Hershey's)	1 oz.	142	17.2
Chocolate-covered (Kraft)	1 piece	14	1.0
Sugar-coated (Blue Diamond)	1 oz.	130	
Almond Cluster (Kraft)	1 piece	63	5.0
(Peter Paul)	1-3/16-oz. pkg.	171	19.8
Almond Joy Peter Paul)	1¾-oz. pkg.	231	28.1
Almond Toffee Bar (Kraft)	1 oz.	142	17.9
Babies, Chocolate flavor (Heide)	1 oz.	101	
Baby Ruth (Curtiss)	1 oz.	135	21.0
Berries (Mason)	1 oz.	100	
Black Crows (Mason)	1 oz.	100	
Brazil nuts, Chocolate-covered (Kraft)	1 piece	32	1.7

C
D

Food and Description	Measure or Quantity	Calories	Carbohydrates (grams)
Bridge Mix, Almond (Kraft)	1 piece	22	1.6
Caramelette (Kraft)	1 piece	12	1.9
Jelly (Kraft)	1 piece	12	2.0
Malted milk ball (Kraft)	1 piece	11	1.4
Mintette (Kraft)	1 piece	12	1.8
Peanut (Kraft)	1 piece	8	.5
Peanut crunch (Kraft)	1 piece	23	3.4
Raisin (Kraft)	1 piece	5	.8
(Nabisco)	1 piece	8	1.4
Butterfinger (Curtiss)	1 oz.	134	21.0
Butternut (Hollywood)	1¼ oz. bar	168	20.6
Butterscotch Skimmers (Nabisco)	1 piece	25	5.7
Candy Corn (Brach's)	1 piece	7	1.8
(Heide)	1 oz.	101	
Caramel (Curtiss)	1 oz.	119	24.1
Chocolate (Kraft)	1 piece	33	6.2
Chocolate bar (Kraft)	1 piece	26	4.9
Chocolate-covered (Brach's)	1 piece	41	7.4
Coconut (Kraft)	1 piece	32	5.5
Milk Duds (Holloway)	1 oz.	111	
Milk Maid (Brach's)	1 piece	34	6.3
Vanilla (Kraft)	1 piece	33	6.2
Vanilla, bar (Kraft)	1 piece	26	4.9
Vanilla, chocolate-covered (Kraft)	1 piece	39	6.2
Vanilla, Twisteroo (Kraft)	1 piece	25	4.7
Caramelette (Kraft)	1 piece	12	1.9
Caravelle (Peter Paul)	1½-oz. pkg.	190	28.5
Carmallow (Queen Anne)	1 piece	83	
Cashew cluster (Kraft)	1 piece	58	4.9
Cashew crunch, canned (Planters)	1 oz.	134	14.4
Charleston Chew, 5¢ size	1 bar (¾ oz.)	90	16.2
10¢ size	1 bar (1-1/8 oz.)	149	26.9
Bite-size	1 piece (7 gr.)	30	5.4

Food and Description	Measure or Quantity	Cal- ories	Carbo- hydrates (grams)
Cherry, Chocolate-covered			
(Brach's)	1 piece	66	13.2
Chocolate-covered, dark			
Welsh's (Nabisco)	1 piece	67	13.0
Chocolate-covered, milk			
Welsh's (Nabisco)	1 piece	66	13.1
Cherry-A-Let (Hoffman)	1 piece	215	
Chewees (Curtiss)	1 oz.	116	24.1
Chocolate Bar, (Nestle's)	1 oz.	148	13.1
Semisweet (Nestle's)	1 oz.	141	17.3
Semisweet Eagel (Ghirandelli)	1 sq.	151	16.7
Special dark, Miniature			
(Hershey's)	1 oz.	145	17.0
(Hershey's)	¼ oz.	37	4.2
With almonds (Nestle's)	1 oz.	149	15.3
(Ghirandelli)	1.1-oz. bar	173	17.6
Milk chocolate (Ghirandelli)	1.1-oz. bar	169	18.9
(Hershey's)	1.05 oz.	150	17
Miniature (Hershey's)	¼ oz.	38	4.0
With almonds (Hershey's)	1.05 oz.	160	15
Mint chocolate bar			
(Ghirandelli)	1.1-oz. bar	171	18.7
Chocolate Block, Milk (Chuckles)	1 oz.	92	23.0
(Chunky)	1 oz.	131	
(Ghirandelli)	1 sq.	147	16.2
(Hershey's)	1 oz.	145	17.8
Circlets (Curtiss)	1 oz.	108	26.1
Circus Peanuts (Brach's)	1 piece	27	6.4
Chocolate Crisp bar (Ghirandelli)	1-oz. bar	161	17.6
(Hershey's)	1 oz.	132	18.6
Chocolate Crunch bar (Nestle's)	1 oz.	140	17.8
Chocolate Parfait (Pearson's)	1 piece	34	
Choc-Shop (Hoffman)	1 piece	241	
Chuckles, Variety pack (Nabisco)	1 piece	41	10.1
	2-oz. pack	206	50.3
Cluster, crispy (Nabisco)	1 piece	65	14.0
Peanut, Chocolate-covered			
(Brach's)	1 piece	79	7.0
(Kraft)	1 piece	59	4.1

Food and Description	Measure or Quantity	Calories	Carbohydrates (grams)
Royal Clusters (Nabisco)	1 piece	78	7.5
Coco-Mello (Nabisco)	1 piece	91	13.8
Coconut, bar (Curtiss)	1 oz.	126	21.0
Welsh's (Nabisco)	1 piece	132	21.8
Bon Bons (Brach's)	1 piece	70	12.6
Cream Egg (Hershey's)	1 oz.	142	20.4
Neopolitan (Brach's)	1 piece	48	8.0
Squares (Nabisco)	1 piece	64	12.3
Coffee-ets (Saylor's)	1 piece	13	
Coffee Nips (Pearson's)	1 piece	26	
Cup-O-Gold (Hoffman)	1 piece	210	
Dots (Mason)	1 oz.	100	
Eggs, Chuckles (Nabisco)	1 piece	10	2.3
Fiddle Faddle	1½-oz. packet	177	34.7
5th Avenue bar, 5¢ size (Luden's)	1 bar	71	
10¢ size (Luden's)	1 bar	129	
15¢ size (Luden's)	1 bar	179	
Frappe, Welsh's (Nabisco)	1 piece	132	23.5
Fruit'n Nut, Chocolate bar (Nestle's)	1 oz.	140	16.5
Fudge, bar, Welsh's (Nabisco)	1 piece	144	25
(Tom Houston)	1 bar	179	29.0
Nut, bars, or squares (Nabisco)	1 piece	71	10.2
Home style (Nabisco)	1 piece	90	13.9
Fudgies, Twisteroo (Kraft)	1 piece	26	4.8
Regular (Kraft)	1 piece	33	6.1
Bar (Kraft)	1 piece	27	5.0
Good & Fruity.	1 oz.	106	26.3
Good & Plenty.	1 oz.	100	24.8
Hard Candy (Bonomo)	1 oz.	112	
(H-B)	1 drop	12	2.9
(Peerless Maid)	1 piece	22	5.6
Butterscotch Disks (Brach's)	1 piece	23	5.7
(Reed's)	1 piece	17	
Cinnamon (Reed's)	1 piece	17	
Lemon drops (Brach's)	1 piece	15	3.8
Peppermint (Reed's)	1 piece	17	

Food and Description	Measure or Quantity	Calories	Carbohydrates (grams)
Pops, assorted (Brach's)	1 piece	19	4.8
Root beer (Reed's)	1 piece	17	
Sherbit (F & F)	1 piece	9	3.2
Sour Balls (Brach's)	1 piece	22	5.7
Spearmint (Reed's)	1 piece	17	
Stix Bars (Jolly Rancher)	1 oz.	102	25.5
Stix Kisses (Jolly Rancher)	1 piece	27	7.0
Stix Pak (Jolly Rancher)	1 piece	18	4.0
Wintergreen (Reed's)	1 piece	17	
Hershey-Ets, Candy-coated	1 oz.	134	21.0
Hollywood	1½-oz. bar	183	28.9
$100,000 Bar (Nestle's)	1 oz.	121	18.9
Jelly Beans (Brach's)	1 piece	11	2.8
(Heide)	1 oz.	90	
Big Bean Jellies (Brach's)	1 piece	26	6.8
Jelly, Iced jelly cones (Brach's)	1 piece	15	3.4
Nougats (Brach's)	1 piece	43	10.0
Rings, Chuckles (Nabisco)	1 piece	37	9.0
Jube Jels (Brach's)	1 piece	11	2.7
Jujubes, assorted (Heide)	1 oz.	93	
Chuckles (Nabisco)	1 piece	13	3.3
Jujufruits (Neide)	1 oz.	94	
Kisses (Hershey's)	1 oz. or 6 pieces	150	15
Kit-Kat.	1¼-oz. bar	171	
Krackel Bar (Hershey's)	1 oz.	148	15.0
Miniature (Hershey's)	¼ oz.	37	3.8
Licorice, Chuckles (Nabisco)	1 piece	36	9.0
Diamond Drops (Heide)	1 oz.	94	
Pastilles (Heide)	1 oz.	96	
Red or black (Switzer)	1 oz.	100	24.0
Twist, Red (American Licorice Co.)	1 piece	33	7.3
Black (American Licorice Co.)	1 piece	27	6.4
Life Savers, Drop (Beech-Nut)	1 piece	10	2.4
Mint (Beech-Nut)	1 piece	7	1.7
Lozenges, mint or wintergreen (Brach's)	1 piece	11	2.9

C
D

Food and Description	Measure or Quantity	Calories	Carbohydrates (grams)
Mallow Cup, 5¢ size (Boyer)	¾ oz.	104	14.8
10¢ size (Boyer)	1¼ oz.	173	24.6
15¢ size (Boyer)	1-5/8 oz.	225	32.3
Malted Milk Balls, Chocolate-covered (Brach's)	1 piece	9	1.6
Malted Milk Crunch (Nabisco)	1 piece	9	.9
Maple Nut goodies (Brach's)	1 piece	29	4.0
Mars Almond bar (M&M/Mars)	1 oz.	130	16.9
Marshmallow (Campfire)	1 oz.	111	24.9
Chocolate (Kraft)	1 piece	24	5.4
Coconut (Kraft)	1 piece	40	7.5
Eggs, Chuckles (Nabisco)	1 piece	38	9.3
Flavored, miniature (Kraft)	1 piece	2	.5
Flavored, regular (Kraft)	1 piece	23	5.8
Royal marshmallow (Curtiss)	1 oz.	90	22.0
White miniature (Kraft)	1 piece	2	.5
White, regular (Kraft)	1 piece	23	5.8
Mary Jane, 1¢ size (Miller)	1 piece (9 gr.)	31	5.6
5¢ size (Miller)	1 piece (1¼ oz.)	125	21.8
Milk Shake (Hollywood)	1¼-oz. bar	148	26.8
Milky Way, dark or milk chocolate (Mars)	1 oz.	120	17.7
Mint or peppermint, Afterdinner, Butter (Richardson)	1 oz.	109	27.0
Colored, pastel (Richardson)	1 oz.	109	28.0
Jelly center (Richardson)	1 oz.	104	26.0
Midget (Richardson)	1 oz.	109	27.0
Striped (Richardson)	1 oz.	109	28.0
Mint or peppermint, Buttermint (Kraft)	1 piece	8	2.0
Chocolate-covered, bar (Brach's)	1 piece	74	13.8
(Richardson's)	1 oz.	106	27.0
Dessert (Brach's)	1 piece	4	.9
Encore (Kraft)	1 piece	6	1.7
Jamaica Mints (Nabisco)	1 piece	24	5.8
Liberty Mints (Nabisco)	1 piece	24	5.8

Food and Description	Measure or Quantity	Calories	Carbohydrates (grams)
Merri-mints (Delson)	1 piece	30	
Mini-mint (Kraft)	1 piece	12	1.9
Mint-Parfait (Pearson's)	1 piece	34	
Party (Kraft)	1 piece	8	2.0
Pattie chocolate-covered (Brach's)	1 piece	50	9.2
(Mason Mints)	1 oz.	200	
Junior Mint Pattie (Nabisco)	1 piece	10	2.0
Peppermint pattie (Nabisco)	1 piece	64	12.5
Sherbit, pressed mints (F&F)	1 piece	7	1.8
Starlight Mints (Brach's)	1 piece	19	4.8
Swedish (Brach's)	1 piece	8	1.9
Thin (Delson)	1 piece	45	
(Nabisco)	1 piece	42	8.1
Wafers (Nabisco)	1 piece	10	1.0
Mounds (Peter Paul)	1-9/10-oz. pkg.	236	31.1
M&M's, Plain chocolate (M&M/Mars)	1 oz.	140	18.1
Peanut (M&M/Mars)	1 oz.	140	16.8
Mr. Goodbar (Hershey's)	1.3 oz.	210	18
Miniature (Hershey's)	¼ oz.	38	3.2
Canada Mints (Necco)	1 piece	13	
Necco Wafers (Necco)	1 piece	7	
Nibs. Cherry (Y&S)	1¾ oz.	179	40.0
Licorice (Y&S)	1¾ oz.	179	40.0
North Pole (F&F)	1-3/8-oz. bar	150	31.0
Nougat centers, Chuckles (Nabisco)	1 piece	17	4.2
Nutty Crunch (Nabisco)	1 piece	71	10.2
Orange slices (Brach's)	1 piece	55	14.4
Chuckles (Nabisco)	1 piece	29	7.2
Payday (Hollywood)	1¼-oz. bar	154	22.3
Peaks (Mason)	1 oz.	175	
Peanut, Chocolate-covered, Candy-coated (Hershey's)	1 oz.	139	17.9
Chocolate-coated (Kraft)	1 piece	12	.9

Food and Description	Measure or Quantity	Calories	Carbohydrates (grams)
Chocolate-covered (Nabisco)	1 piece	24	1.6
(B&B)	1 oz.	158	6.5
(Brach's)	1 piece	11	1.1
Peanut, French Burnt (Brach's)	1 piece	5	.6
Peanut Brittle (Kraft)	1 oz.	126	19.8
(Bonomo)	1 oz.	132	
Jumbo Peanut Block bar (Planter's)	1 oz.	139	14.0
Coconut (Kraft)	1 oz.	125	21.7
Peanut Butter Cup, 5¢ size (Boyer)	¾ oz.	130	10.8
10¢ size (Boyer)	1¼ oz.	216	17.9
15¢ size (Boyer)	1-5/8 oz.	281	23.6
Smoothie, 5¢ size (Boyer)	¾ oz.	135	10.8
10¢ size (Boyer)	1¼ oz.	224	17.9
15¢ size (Boyer)	1-5/8 oz.	292	23.6
(Reese's)	1.2 oz.	190	18
(Reese's)	1 oz.	143	15.4
Peanut Butter Egg (Reese's)	1 oz.	133	12.4
P-Nut Butter Crunch (Pearson's)	1 piece	35	
Pom Poms (Nabisco)	1 piece	14	2.3
Poppycock.	1 oz.	147	22.0
Raisin, Chocolate-covered (Nabisco)	1 piece	4	.6
(Brach's)	1 piece	4	.7
Raisinets (BB)	5¢-size pkg.	140	15.4
Red Hot Dollars (Heide)	1 oz.	94	
Saf-T-Pops (Curtiss)	1 oz.	108	26.1
Screaming Yellow Zonkers.	1 oz.	120	23.1
Snickers (M&M/Mars)	1 oz.	130	15.0
Spearmint leaves (Brach's)	1 piece	23	5.9
Chuckles (Nabisco)	1 piece	27	6.6
Spice flavored sticks & drops, Chuckles (Nabisco)	1 piece	13	3.4
Spice flavored strings, Chuckles (Nabisco)	1 piece	18	4.6
Spicettes (Brach's)	1 piece	10	2.5

Food and Description	Measure or Quantity	Calories	Carbohydrates (grams)
Sprigs, sweet chocolate			
(Hershey's)	1 oz.	136	18.3
Stars, chocolate (Brach's)	1 piece	16	1.7
(Kraft)	1 piece	13	1.5
(Nabisco)	1 piece	15	1.6
Sugar Babies (Nabisco)	1 piece	6	1.3
Sugar Daddy, caramel sucker,			
(Nabisco)	1 piece	121	26.4
Junior (Nabisco)	1 piece	50	11.1
Junior, Choco-flavored			
(Nabisco)	1 piece	51	10.6
Nugget (Nabisco)	1 piece	48	10.5
	(4 oz.)		
(Nabisco)	1 piece	27	6.0
Sugar Mama (Nabisco)	1 piece	101	18.6
Sugar Wafer (F&F)	1¼-oz.	180	26.0
	pkg.		
Taffy, assorted (Brach's)	1 piece	28	5.2
Chocolate (Kraft)	1 piece	27	5.1
Coffee (Kraft)	1 piece	28	5.2
Rum butter (Kraft)	1 piece	28	5.2
Salt-water (Brach's)	1 piece	31	6.8
Turkish, bar (Bonomo)	5¢ size	115	29.3
	(1-1/8 oz.)		
Miniatures (Bonomo)	1 piece	21	5.6
Nibbles, chocolate-covered			
(Bonomo)	1 piece	9	1.6
Pop (Bonomo)	1 piece	45	11.3
Roll (Bonomo)	1¢ size	21	5.6
Vanilla (Kraft)	1 piece	28	5.2
3 Musketeers (M&M/Mars)	1 oz.	120	19.6
Tootsie Roll, Regular, Vending			
machine size:	1 piece	21	3.9
1¢ size or midget.	1 piece	26	5.0
2¢ size.	1 piece	43	8.1
5¢ size.	1 piece	87	16.2
10¢ size.	1 piece	174	32.3
Twin pak, 10¢ size.	1¼ oz.	137	26.9
15¢ size.	2 oz.	219	43.1

C
D

Food and Description	Measure or Quantity	Calories	Carbohydrates (grams)
Tootsie Roll, Pop, 2 for 5¢	1 piece (.5 oz.)	18	4.4
Pop 5¢ size.	1 piece (5 gr.)	110	26.4
Triple Decker bar *(Nestle's)*	1 oz.	148	16.8
Twizzlers, chocolate *(Y&S)*	1 oz.	102	22.0
Grape *(Y&S)*	1 oz.	96	23.0
Licorice *(Y&S)*	1¾ oz.	172	40.0
Strawberry *(Y&S)*	1¾-oz. bar	168	40.0
Strawberry *(Y&S)*	1-oz. bar	96	23.0
Virginia Nut Roll *(Queen Anne)*	10¢ size	250	
Walnut Hill *(F&F)*	1-3/8-oz. bar	177	29.0
Whirligigs *(Nabisco)*	1 piece	26	5.1
Wetem & Wearem *(Heide)*	1 oz.	94	
Wintergreen *(Necco)*	1 piece	13	
CANDY—DIETETIC			
Almonds, Chocolate-covered *(Estee)*	1 piece	22	1.6
Chocolate bar, Bittersweet *(Estee)*	1 bar (¾ oz.)	125	8.9
(Estee)	1 section 2-oz. bar	14	1.0
(Estee)	1 section 4-oz. bar	83	5.9
Coconut *(Estee)*	1 bar (¾ oz.)	124	8.5
Crunch *(Estee)*	1 bar (5/8 oz.)	101	8.6
(Estee)	1 section 3-oz. bar	61	5.1
Fruit-nut *(Estee)*	1 section 4-oz. bar	81	6.6
Milk chocolate *(Estee)*	1 bar (¾ oz.)	126	9.4
(Estee)	1 section 2 oz. bar	14	1.0

Food and Description	Measure or Quantity	Calories	Carbohydrates (grams)
(Estee)	1 section 4-oz. bar	84	6.2
Peppermint (Estee)	1 bar (¾ oz.)	126	9.4
White (Estee)	1 section 4-oz. bar	79	6.1
Almonds (Estee)	1 bar (¾ oz.)	125	8.9
(Estee)	1 section 2-oz. bar	14	1.0
(Estee)	1 section 4-oz. bar	83	5.9
Chocolates, Assorted, milk (Estee)	1 piece	50	3.3
Slimtreats (Estee)	1 piece	13	1.3
Chocolettes, Milk or peppermint (Estee)	1 piece	18	1.5
Creams, Assorted or peppermint (Estee)	1 piece	49	3.4
Gum Drops, Assorted & cherry (Estee)	1 piece	3	.8
Gum Drops, Licorice (Estee)	1 piece	2	.6
Hard candy, Assorted, Cherry & lemon (Estee)	1 piece	12	3.0
Coffee (Estee)	1 piece	12	2.8
Licorice (Estee)	1 piece	12	3.0
Lolly pop (Estee)	1 pop	12	3.0
Mint, any flavor (Estee)	1 piece	4	1.0
Peppermint (Estee)	1 piece	12	3.0
Slimtreats	1 piece	9	2.5
Nut, Chocolate-covered (Estee)	1 piece	48	3.2
Peanut butter cup, (Estee)	1 piece	42	2.5
Peanut, Chocolate-covered (Estee)	1 piece	7	.5
Petit fours (Estee)	1 piece	48	2.5
Raisin, Chocolate-covered (Estee)	1 piece	5	.7
TV mix (Estee)	1 piece	11	.8

C
D

CEREALS

Food and Description	Measure or Quantity	Calories	Carbo-hydrates (grams)
Alpha-Bits *(Post)*	1 cup	110	24
Bran, All-bran, Wheat bran			
Cereal *(Kellogg's)*	1 oz.	60	20
100% Bran cereal *(Nabisco)*	½ cup	70	21
Raisin bran *(Kellogg's)*	1 oz.	100	31
(Post)	1 oz.	100	22
Bran buds *(Kellogg's)*	1 oz.	70	21
Bran cereal, Total, bran			
cereal *(General Mills)*	1 oz.	110	23
Bran flakes, 40% *(Kellogg's)*	1 oz.	70	22
40% *(Post)*	1 oz.	100	22
40% bran, added thiamin & iron *(USDA)*	1 cup	105	28
With raisins, added thiamin & iron *(USDA)*	1 cup	145	40
Cocoa Puffs *(General Mills)*	1 oz.	110	25
Corn cereal, Golden Grahams *(General Mills)*	1 oz.	110	24
Honeycomb crisp sweetened corn cereal *(Post)*	1 oz.	110	25
Kix corn cereal *(General Mills)*	1 oz.	110	24
Sugarpops, puffed corn *(Kellogg's)*	1 oz.	110	26
Trix corn cereal *(General Mills)*	1 oz.	110	25
Corn Total *(General Mills)*	1 oz.	110	24
Corn flakes, Country corn flakes *(General Mills)*	1 oz.	110	24
(Kellogg's)	1 oz.	110	25
Post Toasties *(Post)*	1 oz.	110	24
Corn flakes, added nutrients, plain *(USDA)*	1 cup	100	21
Corn flakes, sugar-covered *(USDA)*	1 cup	155	36
Sugar Frosted flakes *(Kellogg's)*	1 oz.	110	26

Food and Description	Measure or Quantity	Calories	Carbohydrates (grams)
Corn flake crumbs (Kellogg's)	1 oz.	110	25
Corn (hominy) grits, degermed, cooked, enriched (USDA)	1 cup	125	27
Enriched hominy grits, cooked (Quaker or Aunt Jemina)	2/3 cup	100	22
unenriched (USDA)	1 cup	125	27
Instant grits product (Quaker)	1 packet	78	17.5
Farina, Enriched (H-O Cream)	2 tbsp. dry	80	17
(Quaker)	1/6 cup uncooked	100	22.1
Quick cooking, enriched, cooked (USDA)	1 cup	105	22
Granola, Nature Valley, cinnamon & raison (General Mills)	1 oz.	130	19
Grape-nuts flakes (Post)	1 oz.	100	23
Lucky Charms (General Mills)	1 oz.	110	24
Oats, With or without corn, Puffed, added nutrients (USDA)	1 cup	100	19
Cheerios, oat cereal (General Mills)	1 oz.	110	20
Frosty O's (General Mills)	1 oz.	110	24
Old fashioned oats (H-O)	½ cup dry	140	24
Quick oats (H-O)	½ cup dry	130	23
Quick or old fashioned oats (Quaker)	⅓ cup uncooked	107	18.8
Oat flakes, fortified (Post)	1 oz.	110	20
Oatmeal, or rolled oats, cooked (USDA)	1 cup	130	23
Instant oatmeal (H-O)	½ cup dry	130	23
Rice, Cocoa Crispies, oven toasted rice cereal (Kellogg's)	1 oz.	110	26
Frosted rice cereal (Kellogg's)	1 oz.	110	26
Rice Krinkles, frosted (Post)	1 oz.	110	26
Rice Krispies (Kellogg's)	1 oz.	110	25
Puffed rice (Quaker)	1 cup	56	12.5
Puffed rice, added nutrients (USDA)	1 cup	60	13

C
D

Food and Description	Measure or Quantity	Calories	Carbohydrates (grams)
Wheat, Buc Wheats (General Mills)	1 oz.	110	23
Cream of Wheat, regular (Nabisco)	2½ tbsp.	100	22
Quick (Nabisco)	2½ tbsp.	100	21
Pep, wheat flakes (Kellogg's)	1 oz.	100	24
Wheat flakes, added nutrients (USDA)	1 cup	105	24
Puffed wheat (Quaker)	1 cup	51	11.2
Puffed wheat, added nutrients (USDA)	1 cup	55	12
Shredded wheat biscuit (Nabisco)	1 biscuit	80	17
Shredded wheat (Quaker)	2 biscuits	135	28.7
Plain (USDA)	1 biscuit	90	20
Spoon size shredded wheat (Nabiscc)	⅔ cup	110	23
Sugar Smacks, wheat cereal (Kellogg's)	1 oz.	110	25
Wheaties, whole wheat cereal (USDA)	1 oz.	100	23
CHEESE			
American or Cheddar, Natural (USDA)	1 oz.	115	1
	1 cu. in.	70	Trace
Natural (Foremost Blue Moon)	1-oz. slice	100	Trace
(Kraft)	1 oz.	113	.6
Natural, Cheddar (Sealtest)	1 oz.	115	.6
Natural, grated (Kraft)	1 oz.	129	8.4
Natural, grated or shredded (USDA)	1 cup	442	2.3
(USDA)	1 tbsp.	27	.1
Natural, Sharp cheddar (Wispride)	1 tbsp.	50	1.5
Natural, shredded (Kraft)	1 oz.	113	.6
American, Pasteurized processed (USDA)	1 oz.	105	1
(USDA)	1 cu. in.	65	Trace

Food and Description	Measure or Quantity	Calories	Carbo-hydrates (grams)
American or cheddar, Processed			
(USDA)	1 oz.	105	.5
(Borden)	1-oz. slice	106	.9
(Borden)	¾-oz. slice	79	.7
Cheddar, regular (Borden)	1 oz.	113	.6
Dried, sharp cheddar (Data from General Mills Laboratory)	1 oz.	171	1.7
Grated (Borden)	1 tbsp.	30	.1
Loaf or slice (Kraft)	1 oz.	105	.5
Longhorn (Borden)	1 oz.	113	.6
Made in Wisconsin (Borden)	1 oz.	104	.6
Vera Sharp (Borden)	1 oz.	104	.6
Wisconsin old fashioned (Borden)	1 oz.	113	.6
American, Processed (USDA)	1-oz. slice 3½ × 3-3/8 × 1/8 in.	92	2.0
	1-in. cube (.6 oz.)	58	1.3
	1 tbsp. (.5 oz.)	45	1.0
(Borden)	1-oz. slice	93	2.3
(Foremost Blue Moon)	1 oz.	87	1.5
Grated (Borden)	1 oz.	134	11.0
Grated (Used in Kraft Dinner)	1 oz.	129	8.4
Slices (Kraft)	1 oz.	94	2.4
Slices, Cheez'n bacon (Kraft)	1 oz.	101	1.1
Links, Bacon, Handi-Snack (Kraft)	1 oz.	93	2.2
Links, Garlic, Handi-Snack (Kraft)	1 oz.	92	2.2
Links, Jalapeño, Handi-Snack (Kraft)	1 oz.	92	2.2
Links, Nippy, Handi-Snack (Kraft)	1 oz.	92	2.2
Links, Smokelle, Handi-Snack (Kraft)	1 oz.	93	2.2

C
D

73

Food and Description	Measure or Quantity	Calories	Carbohydrates (grams)
Links, Swiss, Handi-Snack (Kraft)	1 oz.	90	1.4
Loaf, Munst-ett (Kraft)	1 oz.	100	1.7
Loaf, Pizzalone (Kraft)	1 oz.	90	.5
Loaf, Super blend (Kraft)	1 oz.	92	1.6
Pimento (Borden)	1 oz.	91	2.0
Pimento slices (Kraft)	1 oz.	94	2.5
Salami slices (Kraft)	1 oz.	94	2.6
Swiss (Borden)	1 oz.	92	1.7
Swiss, slices (Kraft)	1 oz.	92	2.3
Blue or Roquefort, natural type (USDA)	1 oz.	105	1
	1-cu. in.	65	Trace
Bleu or Blue, Natural, crumbled (USDA)	1 cup	497	2.7
(Foremost Blue Moon)	1 tbsp.	52	Trace
(Frigo)	1 oz.	99	.5
Natural (Kraft)	1 oz.	99	.5
(Stella)	1 oz.	112	.6
(Wispride)	2 tbsp. (1 oz.)	98	3.2
Blufort (Borden)	1¼-oz. pkg.	131	.7
Danish (Borden)	1 oz.	105	.6
Flora Danica (Borden)	1 oz.	105	.6
Bondost, Natural (Kraft)	1 oz.	103	.4
Brick, Natural (USDA)	1 oz.	105	.5
(Borden)	1 oz.	105	.5
(Kraft)	1 oz.	103	.3
Process, slices (Kraft)	1 oz.	101	.4
Camembert, Domestic, natural (USDA)	1 oz.	85	.5
Packaged in 4-oz. pkg. with 3 wedges per pkg. (USDA)	1 wedge	114	.7
(Borden)	1 oz.	86	.5
Natural (Kraft)	1 oz.	85	.5
Caraway, Natural (Kraft)	1 oz.	111	.6
Casino Swiss, Natural (Kraft)	1 oz.	104	.5
Chantelle, Natural (Kraft)	1 oz.	90	.3

Food and Description	Measure or Quantity	Calories	Carbohydrates (grams)
Cheez-ola, Process (Fisher)	1 oz.	90	1.1
Colby, Natural (Borden)	1 oz.	111	.6
(Kraft)	1 oz.	111	.6
Cottage, large or small curd, Creamed, partially (Meadow Gold)	1 cup	204	6.0
Creamed, unflavored (USDA)	1 oz.	30	.8
(USDA)	8-oz. pkg.	240	6.6
(Borden)	8-oz. container	240	6.6
(Foremost Blue Moon)	1 oz.	30	.4
(Kraft)	1 oz.	27	.9
(Meadow Gold)	1 cup	234	6.0
(Sealtest)	1 cup	213	4.7
California (Breakstone)	8-oz. container	216	4.8
California (Breakstone)	1 tbsp.	15	.3
Light'n Lively (Sealtest)	1 cup	155	5.6
Lite Line (Borden)	1 cup	189	7.0
Low fat, 2% fat (Sealtest)	1 cup	193	7.4
Made with raw non-fat milk (Alta-Dena)	1 cup	232	
Cottage, Stay'N Shape Lowfat	4 oz.	92	3.5
(Breakstone)	8 oz.	184	7.9
	1 tbsp.	13	.6
Tangy Small Curd	4 oz.	108	2.1
(Breakstone)	8 oz.	216	4.8
	1 tbsp.	15	.3
Cottage, Creamed, unflavored, tiny soft curd (Breakstone)	8 oz.	216	4.8
	1 tbsp.	15	.3
Cottage, Creamed, flavored, Chive (Breakstone)	8-oz. container	216	4.8
	1 tbsp.	15	.3
(Sealtest)	1 cup	211	4.7
Chive-pepper (Sealtest)	1 cup	206	5.4
Peach, low fat			

C
D

Food and Description	Measure or Quantity	Calories	Carbohydrates (grams)
(Breakstone)	8-oz. container	232	24.9
	1 tbsp.	17	1.8
Peach-pineapple (Sealtest)	1 cup	228	17.9
Pineapple, low fat (Breakstone)	8-oz. container	268	34.2
	1 tbsp.	19	2.4
Pineapple (Sealtest)	1 cup	222	16.1
Spring Garden Salad (Sealtest)	1 cup	208	67
Cottage, large or small curd, Creamed, curd press down (USDA)	1 cup	260	7.1
Uncreamed, curd pressed down (USDA)	1 cup	170	5
	8-oz. pkg.	195	6.1
	1 oz.	24	.8
Uncreamed (Foremost Blue Moon)	1 oz.	30	.2
(Sealtest)	1 cup	179	1.6
Pot, unsalted (Borden)	8-oz. pkg.	195	6.1
Cottage, Pot Style (Breakstone)	4 oz.	86	1.7
	8-oz. container	172	3.9
Skim Milk (Breakstone)	4 oz.	91	.7
	8-oz. container	182	1.6
	1 tbsp.	13	.1
Country Charm, Natural (Fisher)	1 oz.	89	.4
4% Milkfat Min. (Meadow Gold)	½ cup	120	4
2% Milkfat, Viva Lowfat (Meadow Gold)	½ cup	100	4
Cream Cheese, Package of 3 oz. net wt. (USDA)	1 pkg.	320	2
Package of 8 oz. net wt. (USDA)	1 pkg.	850	5
Plain, unwhipped (USDA)	1 oz.	106	.6

Food and Description	Measure or Quantity	Cal- ories	Carbo- hydrates (grams)
(USDA)	1-in. cube	60	.3
(Borden)	1 oz.	96	.6
(Breakstone)	1 oz.	98	.6
	1 tbsp.	49	.3
(Kraft)	1 oz.	104	.9
(Sealtest)	1 oz.	98	.6
Cream Cheese, Plain, unwhipped, Hostess (Kraft)	1 oz.	98	.6
Philadelphia (Kraft)	1 oz.	104	.9
Philadelphia, Imitation (Kraft)	1 oz.	52	1.9
Cream Cheese, Temp-Tee Whipped (Breakstone)	1 oz.	98	2.0
	1 tbsp.	32	.2
Cream Cheese, Flavored, Unwhipped, Chive (Borden)	1 oz.	96	.6
Chive, Hostess (Kraft)	1 oz.	84	.8
Chive, Philadelphia (Kraft)	1 oz.	84	.8
Date & nut (Borden)	1 oz.	96	
Olive-pimento, Hostess (Kraft)	1 oz.	84	.8
Pimento (Borden)	1 oz.	74	.6
Pimento, Hostess (Kraft)	1 oz.	85	.7
Pimento, Philadelphia (Kraft)	1 oz.	85	.7
Pineapple, Hostess (Kraft)	1 oz.	86	2.5
Roquefort, Hostess (Kraft)	1 oz.	80	.7
Cream Cheese, Flavored, whipped Bacon & horseradish (Kraft)	1 oz.	96	.7
Blue (Kraft)	1 oz.	97	1.2
Catalina (Kraft)	1 oz.	94	1.1
Chive (Kraft)	1 oz.	92	1.0
Onion (Kraft)	1 oz.	93	1.5
Pimento (Kraft)	1 oz.	91	1.2
Salami (Kraft)	1 oz.	88	1.2
Smoked salmon (Kraft)	1 oz.	90	1.7
Edam (House of Gold)	1 oz.	105	.3
Natural (Kraft)	1 oz.	104	.3
Midget Farmer Cheese (Breakstone)	2 oz.	80	2.1
	1-cu. in.	60	Trace

Food and Description	Measure or Quantity	Calories	Carbohydrates (grams)
Fontina, Natural (Kraft)	1 oz.	113	.6
(Stella)	1 oz.	112	.6
Frankenmuth, Natural (Kraft)	1 oz.	113	.7
Gjetost, Natural (Kraft)	1 oz.	134	13.0
Gorganzola (Foremost Blue Moon)	1 oz.	110	Trace
Natural (Kraft)	1 oz.	111	.4
Gouda, Dutch Maid (Borden)	1 oz.	86	.5
Baby Gouda (Foremost Blue Moon)	1 oz.	120	Trace
Natural (Kraft)	1 oz.	107	.5
Gruyère (Borden)	1 oz.	101	.5
Natural (Kraft)	1 oz.	110	.6
Swiss Knight	1 oz.	101	.5
Jack-dry, Natural (Kraft)	1 oz.	101	.4
Jack-fresh, Natural (Kraft)	1 oz.	95	.4
Lager-Kase, Natural (Kraft)	1 oz.	107	.3
Leyden, Natural (Kraft)	1 oz.	80	.7
Liederkranz (Borden)	1 oz.	86	.4
Limburger, Natural (USDA)	1 oz.	98	.6
(Kraft)	1 oz.	98	.6
Process, Dutch Maid (Borden)	1 oz.	97	.6
Monterey Jack (Borden)	1 oz.	103	.6
(Frigo)	1 oz.	103	.4
Natural (Kraft)	1 oz.	102	.4
Mozzarella, Process (Borden)	1 oz.	96	.8
(Frigo)	1 oz.	79	.3
Low moisture, part skim, Natural (Kraft)	1 oz.	84	.3
Low moisture, part skim, pizza, Natural (Kraft)	1 oz.	79	.3
Shredded (Kraft)	1 oz.	79	.3
Muenster, Natural (Borden)	1 oz.	85	.7
(Kraft)	1 oz.	100	.3
Process, slices (Kraft)	1 oz.	102	.6
Neufchâtel, Natural, Calorie-Wise (Kraft)	1 oz.	70	.7
Process (Borden)	1 oz.	73	6.5
Nuworld, Natural (Kraft)	1 oz.	103	.7

Food and Description	Measure or Quantity	Calories	Carbohydrates (grams)
Old English, Process, Loaf or slices *(Kraft)*	1 oz.	105	.5
Parmesan, Natural *(USDA)*	1 oz.	111	.8
(Frigo)	1 oz.	107	.8
(Kraft)	1 oz.	107	.8
(Sierra)	1 oz.	103	.9
Grated, natural *(USDA)*	1 oz.	130	1
Grated, natural, cup loosely-packed *(USDA)*	1 cup	494	3.6
Cup pressed down *(USDA)*	1 cup	655	5
Grated, natural *(USDA)*	1 tbsp.	25	Trace
(Borden)	1 oz.	143	8.8
(Buitoni)	1 oz.	118	.8
(Frigo)	1 tbsp.	27	.2
(Kraft)	1 oz.	127	1.0
Shredded *(Kraft)*	1 oz.	114	.9
Parmesan & Romano, Grated *(Borden)*	1 oz.	143	.9
	1 tbsp.	31	.2
(Kraft)	1 oz.	130	1.0
Pepata *(Frigo)*	1 oz.	110	.8
Pimento American, Process *(USDA)*	1 oz.	105	.5
(Borden)	1 oz.	104	.5
Loaf or slices *(Kraft)*	1 oz.	103	.4
Made in Wisconsin *(Borden)*	1 oz.	104	.5
Pinconning, Natural *(Kraft)*	1 oz.	113	.7
Pizza *(Borden)*	1 oz.	85	.8
(Frigo)	1 oz.	73	.3
Low fat, part skim, shredded *(Kraft)*	1 oz.	86	.4
Port du Salut *(Foremost Blue Moon)*	1 oz.	100	Trace
Natural *(Kraft)*	1 oz.	100	.3
Primost, Natural *(Kraft)*	1 oz.	134	13.0
Provolone *(Borden)*	1 oz.	93	1.0
Natural *(Kraft)*	1 oz.	99	.5

Food and Description	Measure or Quantity	Calories	Carbohydrates (grams)
Ricotta, Moist (Borden)	1 oz.	42	1.0
(Breakstone)	2 oz.	90	4.5
	1 tbsp.	25	.7
Natural (Kraft)	1 oz.	47	1.3
(Sierra)	1 oz.	50	1.3
Romano, Italian pecorino			
(Borden)	1 oz.	114	.8
(Frigo)	1 oz.	110	.8
Natural (Stella)	1 oz.	106	.6
Grated (Borden)	1 oz.	136	12.1
(Buitoni)	1 oz.	123	1.1
(Frigo)	1 tbsp.	29	.2
(Kraft)	1 oz.	134	1.0
Shredded (Kraft)	1 oz.	121	.9
Romano & Parmesan, Plain			
(Kraft)	1 oz.	133	1.0
Flavored, Bacon smoke			
(Kraft)	1 oz.	130	1.1
Flavored, Garlic (Kraft)	1 oz.	134	1.0
Flavored, Onion (Kraft)	1 oz.	134	1.0
Roquefort, Natural (USDA)	1 oz.	104	.6
Napoleon (Borden)	1 oz.	107	.6
Natural (Kraft)	1 oz.	105	.5
Sage, Natural (Kraft)	1 oz.	113	.6
Sap Sago, Natural (Kraft)	1 oz.	76	1.7
Sardo Romano, Natural (Kraft)	1 oz.	109	.8
Scamorze (Frigo)	1 oz.	79	.3
Natural (Kraft)	1 oz.	100	.3
Special cure, Process, slices			
(Kraft)	1 oz.	105	.5
Supercure, Process, slices			
(Kraft)	1 oz.	105	.5
Swiss, Domestic, Natural			
(USDA)	1 oz.	105	.5
(USDA)	1-cu. in.	55	Trace
(USDA)	1¼-oz. slice (7½ × 4 × 1/16 in.)	130	.6

Food and Description	Measure or Quantity	Calories	Carbo-hydrates (grams)
(Borden)	1 oz.	104	.5
(Foremost Blue Moon)	1 oz.	105	1.0
(Kraft)	1 oz.	104	.5
(Sealtest)	1 oz.	105	.5
(USDA)	1 oz.	100	1
(USDA)	1-cu. in.	65	Trace
Process (Borden)	1-oz. slice	96	.9
	¾-oz. slice	74	.7
Process, Made in Wisconsin			
(Borden)	1 oz.	100	.5
Process, Milk bay (Borden)	1 oz.	96	.5
Process, Smoke-flavored			
(Borden)	1 oz.	103	.5
Process, Loaf (Kraft)	1 oz.	92	.5
Process, slices (Kraft)	1 oz.	95	.6
Process, loaf with Muenster			
(Kraft)	1 oz.	98	.6
Swiss, Imported, natural,			
Finland import (Borden)	1 oz.	104	.5
Switzerland import (Borden)	1 oz.	104	.5
Washed curd, Natural (Kraft)	1 oz.	107	.6

CHEESE SPREAD

Food and Description	Measure or Quantity	Calories	Carbo-hydrates (grams)
American, Process (USDA)	1 oz.	82	2.3
	1 tbsp.	40	1.1
(Borden)	1 oz.	82	2.3
Shredded (USDA)	1 packed cup (4 oz.)	325	9.3
Vera Sharp (Borden)	1 oz.	80	.3
Swankyswig (Kraft)	1 oz.	77	1.7
Snack Mate (Nabisco)	1 tsp.	15	.4
Bacon, cheese'n bacon (Borden)	1 oz.	80	1.2
Bacon, Squeez-A-Snak (Kraft)	1 oz.	83	.5
Bacon, Swankyswig (Kraft)	1 oz.	92	.6
Blue, Process (Borden)	1 oz.	82	2.3
Vera Blue (Borden)	1 oz.	91	.6
Cheddar, Process, Snack Mate			
(Nabisco)	1 tsp.	15	.4

81

Food and Description	Measure or Quantity	Calories	Carbohydrates (grams)
Seasoned, Snack Mate (Nabisco)	1 tsp.	15	.5
Cheez Whiz, Process (Kraft)	1 oz.	76	1.7
Count Down (Fisher)	1 oz.	76	1.7
Garlic, Process (Borden)	1 oz.	82	2.3
Squeeze-A-Snak (Kraft)	1 oz.	84	.5
Swankyswig (Kraft)	1 oz.	86	1.8
Hickory Smoke, Process (Borden)	1 oz.	80	1.3
Snack Mate (Nabisco)	1 tsp.	14	.5
Imitation, Process, Calorie-Wise (Kraft)	1 oz.	48	3.6
Chef's Delight (Fisher)	1 oz.	41	3.4
Mellow Age (Fisher)	1 oz.	41	3.4
Jalapeño, Process, Cheeze Whiz (Kraft)	1 oz.	76	1.9
Limburger (Kraft)	1 oz.	69	.4
Process (Borden)	1 oz.	82	2.3
Neufchâtel, Bacon & horseradish, Party Snacks (Kraft)	1 oz.	74	.7
Chipped beef, Party Snacks (Kraft)	1 oz.	67	1.2
Chive, Party Snacks (Kraft)	1 oz.	69	.8
Clam, Party Snacks (Kraft)	1 oz.	67	.8
Olive-pimento (Borden)	1 oz.	81	2.7
Olive-pimento, Swankyswig (Kraft)	1 oz.	70	1.2
Onion, Party Snacks (Kraft)	1 oz.	66	1.6
Pimento (Borden)	1 oz.	82	2.9
Pimento, Party Snacks (Kraft)	1 oz.	67	1.4
Pimento, Swankyswig (Kraft)	1 oz.	67	1.4
Pineapple (Borden)	1 oz.	81	3.1
Pineapple, Swankyswig (Kraft)	1 oz.	70	2.7
Relish (Borden)	1 oz.	81	3.5
Relish, Swankyswig (Kraft)	1 oz.	71	3.3
Roka, Swankyswig (Kraft)	1 oz.	80	.6
Old English, Process, Swankyswig (Kraft)	1 oz.	96	.6
Onion, French, Process, Snack Mate (Nabisco)	1 tsp.	15	.4

Food and Description	Measure or Quantity	Calories	Carbo-hydrates (grams)
Pimento, Cheez Whiz *(Kraft)*	1 oz.	76	1.7
Process, Squeeze-A-Snak *(Kraft)*	1 oz.	86	.6
Process, Snack Mate *(Nabisco)*	1 tsp.	15	.4
(Sealtest)	1 oz.	77	1.7
Process, Velveeta *(Kraft)*	1 oz.	84	2.6
Sharp, Process, Squeeze-A-Snak *(Kraft)*	1 oz.	85	.6
Sharpie, Process *(Kraft)*	1 oz.	90	.5
Smoke, Process, Squeeze-A-Snak *(Kraft)*	1 oz.	83	.5
Smokelle, Process, Swankyswig *(Kraft)*	1 oz.	90	.5
Velva Kreme, Process *(Borden)*	1 oz.	94	1.1
Velvetta, Process *(Kraft)*	1 oz.	84	2.6

CHEESE DIPS

Food and Description	Measure or Quantity	Calories	Carbo-hydrates (grams)
Bacon & horseradish *(Borden)*	1 oz.	79	2.9
(Breakstone)	1 oz.	55	4.3
	2 tbsp.	62	1.3
Teez *(Kraft)*	1 oz.	57	1.6
Ready Dip, Neufchâtel cheese *(Kraft)*	1 oz.	71	.8
Bacon & smoke, Dip'n Dressing *(Sealtest)*	1 oz.	47	1.7
Blue Cheese *(Breakstone)*	1 oz.	60	4.5
	1 tbsp.	32	.7
Heat'N Dip *(Kaukauna Klub)*	1 oz.	57	
Ready Dip, Neufchâtel cheese *(Kraft)*	1 oz.	69	1.6
Teez *(Kraft)*	1 oz.	51	1.3
Dip'n Dressing *(Sealtest)*	1 oz.	49	1.5
Casino, Dip'n Dressing *(Sealtest)*	1 oz.	44	2.1
Cheddar Cheese *(Breakstone)*	1 oz.	60	5.4
Chipped beef, Dip'n Dressing *(Sealtest)*	1 oz.	46	1.8
Clam, Heat 'N Dip *(Kaukauna Klub)*	1 oz.	64	
Ready Dip, Neufchâtel cheese *(Kraft)*	1 oz.	67	1.8
Teez *(Kraft)*	1 oz.	45	1.5

Food and Description	Measure or Quantity	Cal-ories	Carbo-hydrates (grams)
Clam & lobster *(Borden)*	1 oz.	60	1.7
Cucumber & onion *(Breakstone)*	1 oz.	50	5.6
	1 tbsp.	27	.9
Dill Pickle, Ready Dip, Neuf-châtel cheese *(Kraft)*	1 oz.	67	2.4
Garden Sprice *(Borden)*	1 oz.	66	2.1
Garlic, Teez *(Kraft)*	1 oz.	47	1.5
Green Goddess, Teez *(Kraft)*	1 oz.	46	1.5
Imitation Ham & Spice *(Breakstone)*	1 oz.	50	6.4
Jalapeño bean *(Fritos)*	1 oz.	37	4.1
(Gebhardt)	1 oz.	30	4.0
Jalapeño Pepper *(Breakstone)*	1 oz.	50	6.8
Onion, French *(Borden)*	1 oz.	48	1.8
Dip'n Dressing *(Sealtest)*	1 oz.	46	2.2
Teez *(Kraft)*	1 oz.	43	1.5
Heat'N Dip *(Kaukauna Klub)*	1 oz.	75	
(Breakstone)	1 oz.	55	6.2
	1 tbsp.	29	1.0
Ready Dip, Neufchàtel cheese *(Kraft)*	1 oz.	68	2.0
Onion & garlic, Dip'n Dressing *(Sealtest)*	1 oz.	46	2.2
Salami *(Breakstone)*	1 oz.	60	5.7
Shrimp, Heat'N Dip *(Kaukauna Klub)*	1 oz.	53	
Tasty Tartar *(Borden)*	1 oz.	48	1.8
Western Bar-B-Q *(Borden)*	1 oz.	48	1.8
CHEESE FONDUE			
Fondue, Home recipe *(USDA)*	4 oz.	301	11.3
CHEESE SOUFFLÉ			
Cheese Soufflé, Home recipe *(USDA)*	4 oz.	247	7.0
Frozen *(Stouffer's)*	⅓ of 12-oz. pkg.	243	11.7
CHEWING GUM			
Sweetened, Bazooka, bubble, 1¢ size *(USDA)*	1 piece	18	4.5

Food and Description	Measure or Quantity	Calories	Carbohydrates (grams)
Bazooka, bubble, 5¢ size *(USDA)*	1 piece	85	21.2
Beechies	1 tablet	6	1.6
Beech-Nut	1 stick	10	2.3
Beemans	1 stick	9	2.3
Black Jack	1 stick	9	2.3
Chicklets	1 piece	6	1.1
Chicklets, tiny size	5¢-pkg.	65	
Cinnamint	1 stick	10	2.3
Clove	1 stick	9	2.3
Dentyne	1 piece	4	1.2
Doublemint	1 stick	8	2.3
Fruit Punch	1 stick	10	2.3
Juicy Fruit	1 stick	9	2.4
Peppermint *(Clark)*	1 stick	10	2.3
Sour lemon *(Clark)*	1 stick	10	2.3
Spearmint *(Wrigley's)*	1 stick	8	2.2
Teaberry	1 stick	10	2.3
Unsweetened or Dietetic,			
All flavors *(Clark)*	1 stick	7	1.7
(Estee)	1 stick	8	2.0
Bazooka, bubble, sugarless	1 piece	16	Trace
Bubble *(Estee)*	1 piece	3	.6
Care Free *(Beech-Nut)*	1 stick	6	Trace
Peppermint *Amurol*	1 stick	5	1.8

CHINESE FOOD

Food and Description	Measure or Quantity	Calories	Carbohydrates (grams)
Chicken chow mein, canned			
(La Choy) bi-pack	1 cup	118	8.0
Without noodles, home recipe *(USDA)*	4 oz.	116	4.5
Chop Suey, home recipe with meat *(USDA)*	1 cup (8.8 oz.)	300	12.8
With meat, canned *(USDA)*	1 cup (8.8 oz.)	155	10.5
Chicken, canned *(Hung's)*	8 oz.	120	12.4
Egg Roll, Frozen, Chicken *(Chun King)*	½-oz. roll	28	3.2

Food and Description	Measure or Quantity	Calories	Carbo-hydrates (grams)
Frozen, Chicken & mushroom (*Mow Sang*)	1 roll	69	7.0
Frozen, Lobster & meat (*Chun King*)	½-oz. roll	26	3.7
Frozen, Meat & shrimp (*Chun King*)	½-oz. roll	29	3.7
Frozen, Shrimp (*Hung's*)	1 roll	131	15.7

CHINESE DINNER

Food and Description	Measure or Quantity	Calories	Carbo-hydrates (grams)
Beef chow mein, frozen (*Chun King*)	11-oz. dinner	386	47.9
Beef chop suey, frozen (*Chun King*)	11-oz. dinner	310	46.0
Chicken dinner, frozen,			
Meat compartment	7 oz.	133	8.2
Rice compartment	4 oz.	158	30.2
Complete dinner (*Banquet*)	11 oz.	291	38.5
Chicken chow mein, frozen (*Chun King*)	11 oz.	350	48.0
Chop suey, frozen, Complete dinner (*Banquet*)	11 oz.	287	41.8
Egg foo young, frozen (*Chun King*)	11 oz.	340	53.0
Shrimp chow mein, frozen (*Chun King*)	11 oz.	340	50.0
Frozen (*Swanson*)	11 oz.	356	40.9

CONDIMENTS

Food and Description	Measure or Quantity	Calories	Carbo-hydrates (grams)
Capers (*Crosse & Blackwell*)	1 tbsp. (.6 oz.)	6	1.0
Catsup, Regular pack (*USDA*)	½ cup	149	35.8
	1 tbsp.	19	4.6
Regular (*Del Monte*)	1 tbsp.	20	5.2
(*Heinz*)	1 tbsp.	16	3.8
(*Hunt's*)	1 tbsp.	18	5.8
(*Stokely-Van Camp*)	1 tbsp.	19	4.4
Dietetic pack, Low sodium			

Food and Description	Measure or Quantity	Calories	Carbohydrates (grams)
(USDA)	1 tbsp.	19	4.6
(Tillie Lewis)	1 tbsp.	7	1.5
Tomato catsup (Del Monte)	¼ cup	60	16
(Hunt-Wesson)	1 tbsp.	18.2	5.1
(USDA)	1 tbsp.	15	4
(USDA)	1 cup	290	69
Cauliflower, Sweet, pickled			
(Smucker's)	1 bud (.5 oz.)	24	5.5
Chow Chow (Crosse & Blackwell)	1 tbsp.	6	1.0
Sour (USDA)	1 oz.	8	1.2
Sweet (USDA)	1 oz.	33	7.7
Chutney, Major Grey's			
(Crosse & Blackwell)	1 tbsp.	53	13.1
Horseradish, Prepared (Kraft)	1 oz.	3	.4
(USDA)	1 oz.	11	2.7
Cream Style (Kraft)	1 oz.	9	.7
Mustard, Prepared, Brown			
(Heinz)	1 tsp.	8	.5
(USDA)	1 tsp.	8	.5
Spicy (French's)	1 tsp.	6	.5
Regular, diablo or spicy			
(Gulden's)	1 scant tsp.	6	.4
Prepared, German style			
(Kraft)	1 oz.	30	1.7
Prepared (Grey Poupon)	1 tsp.	4	.4
Horseradish (Best Foods)	1 tsp.	5	.4
(French's)	1 tsp.	6	.4
(Kraft)	1 oz.	29	1.6
Prepared, Medford (French's)	1 tsp.	5	.4
Prepared, Onion (French's)	1 tsp.	7	1.1
Prepared, Ring Star (French's)	1 tsp.	4	.4
Prepared, Salad (French's)	1 tsp.	4	.3
Glass or squeeze pack (Kraft)	1 oz.	23	1.7
Plastic squeeze bottle			
(Kraft)	1 oz.	23	1.7
Prepared, Yellow (USDA)	1 tsp.	7	.6

C
D

Food and Description	Measure or Quantity	Calories	Carbohydrates (grams)
(Gulden's)	(1 scant tsp.) ¼-oz. packet	5	.4
(Heinz)	1 tsp.	5	.5
Olives, Greek-style, salt cured, oil-coated, pitted (USDA)	1 oz.	96	2.5
Greek-style, salt cured, oil-coated, With pits, drained (USDA)	1 oz.	33	.4
Green, pitted & drained, Spanish (Mario's)	1 med. olive	6	<.1
Green, pitted & drained (USDA)	1 oz.	33	.4
	1 olive	6	.1
(USDA)	4 med. or 3 extra large or 2 giant	19	.2
Ripe, by variety, pitted & drained, Ascalano, any size (USDA)	1 oz.	37	.7
Ripe, by size, Colossal (Lindsay)	1 olive	13	.3
Extra large (Lindsay)	1 olive	5	.1
Giant (Lindsay)	1 olive	8	.2
Jumbo (Lindsay)	1 olive	10	.2
Large (Lindsay)	1 olive	5	.1
Mammoth (Lindsay)	1 olive	6	.1
Medium (Lindsay)	1 olive	4	1
Select (Lindsay)	1 olive	3	.1
Supercolossal (Lindsay)	1 olive	16	.3
Super supreme (Lindsay)	1 olive	18	.3
Ripe, pitted & drained, Manzanilla, any size (USDA)	1 oz.	37	.7
Ripe, pitted & drained,			

Food and Description	Measure or Quantity	Calories	Carbo-hydrates (grams)
Mission (USDA)	2 large or 3 small (1 oz.)	18 52	.3 .9
Onions, cocktail (Crosse & Black-well)	1 tbsp.	1	.3
Pickles, Bread & butter (Farming's)	100 gms. 14-fl. oz. bottle	45 215	11.5 51.0
Cucumber, fresh or bread & butter (Del Monte)	3 med. pieces	4	1.0
(Heinz)	3 slices	20	4.7
Dill (Del Monte)	1 large pickle	7	1.4
(Heinz)	4-in. pickle	7	1.1
(L & S Dills)	1 large pickle	15	2.0
Baby, fresh pack (Smucker's)	2¾-in. pickle	3	.6
Candied sticks (Smucker's)	4-in. pickle	46	11.2
Hamburger (Heinz)	3 slices	1	.1
Hamburger (Smucker's)	3 slices	2	.3
Fresh-pack (Bond's)	1 spear	2	.2
Processed (Heinz)	3-in. pickle	1	.1
Medium, whole, 3¾ in. long, 1¼ in. diam. (USDA)	1 pickle	10	1
Fresh, sliced 1½ in. diam. ¼ in. thick (USDA)	2 slices	10	3
Gherkin, sweet, small, whole, Approx. 2½ in. long, ¾ in. diam. (USDA)	1 pickle	20	6
Hot mixed (Smucker's)	4 pieces	5	1.0
Hot peppers (Smucker's)	4-in. pepper	10	2.1
Kosher dill (Bond's)	1 pickle	2	.2
(Lutz & Schramm)	1 large pickle	15	2.0

C
D

Food and Description	Measure or Quantity	Calories	Carbohydrates (grams)
Anisette sponge (Stella D'oro)	1 piece	39	10.0
Anisette toast (Stella D'oro)	1 piece	39	7.8
Applesauce, Regular or iced (Sunshine)	1 piece	86	11.9
Arrowroot (Sunshine)	3.7 gr. per biscuit	16	3
Assortment (USDA)	1 oz.	136	20.1
Lady Stella (Stella D'oro)	1 piece	37	5.0
Lady Joan (Sunshine)	1 piece	42	5.8
Lady Joan, Iced (Sunshine)	1 piece	47	6.1
Aunt Sally, Iced (Sunshine)	1 piece	96	19.7
Bana-Bee (Nabisco)	6 pieces (1¾-oz. pkg.)	253	31.4
Big Treat (Sunshine)	1 piece	153	26.6
Bordeaux (Pepperidge Farm)	1 piece	36	5.1
Breakfast Treats (Stella D'oro)	1 piece	99	15.0
Brown edge wafers (Nabisco)	1 piece	28	4.1
Brownie, Junior (Drake's)	2/3-oz. cake	80	10.0
Brownie (Hostess)	1 piece (2 to pkg.)	100	15.5
		200	31
(Tastykake)	1 pkg. (2¼ oz.)	242	34.0
Brownie, Chocolate nut (Pepperidge Farm)	1 piece	54	6.3
Peanut butter (Tastykake)	1 pkg. (1¾ oz.)	239	32.0
Pecan fudge (Keebler)	1 piece	115	13.9
Brownie, Frozen, with nuts & chocolate icing (USDA)	1 oz.	119	17.2
With nuts from home recipe with enriched flour (USDA)	1 brownie	95	10
Brussels (Pepperidge Farm)	1 piece	42	4.6
Butter, Thin, rich (USDA)	1 oz.	130	20.1
(Nabisco)	1 piece	23	3.6
(Sunshine)	1 piece	23	3.5
Buttercup (Keebler)	1 piece	24	3.6

Food and Description	Measure or Quantity	Calories	Carbohydrates (grams)
Sour, Cucumber (Del Monte)	1 large pickle (3.5 oz.)	6	1.1
(USDA)	4-in. pickle (4.8 oz.)	14	2.7
Sour (Heinz)	2-in. pickle	1	.2
Sweet (Del Monte)	1 med. pickle	14	3.5
Candied (Borden)	1 pickle	72	18.1
Candied midgets (Smucker's)	2-in. pickle	14	3.5
Chips (Smucker's)	1 piece	10	2.5
Cucumber, whole (USDA)	1 oz.	41	10.3
Gherkin (Heinz)	2-in. pickle	16	3.9
Mixed (Heinz)	3 pieces	23	5.6
Sticks, Fresh pack (Smucker's)	4-in. stick	29	7.1
Pickle relish, finely chopped, Sweet (USDA)	1 tbsp.	20	5
	½ cup	108	27.0
Tartar Sauce (USDA)	1 tbsp.	75	1
Vinegar (USDA)	1 tbsp.	Trace	1
Cider vinegar (USDA)	½ cup	17	7.1
Distilled vinegar (USDA)	½ cup	14	6.0
	1 tbsp.	2	8
Red or white wine vinegar (Regina)	1 tbsp.	3	5.1
Watermelon Rind (Crosse & Blackwell)	1 tbsp.	38	9.3

COOKIES

Food and Description	Measure or Quantity	Calories	Carbohydrates (grams)
Almond crescent (Nabisco)	1 piece	34	5.0
Almond toast, Mandel (Stella D'oro)	1 piece	49	9.6
Angelica Goodies (Stella D'oro)	1 piece	100	14.6
Anginetti (Stella D'oro)	1 piece	28	2.4
Animal Cracker (USDA)	1 oz.	122	22.7
Barnum's (Nabisco)	1 piece	12	2.0
Regular (Sunshine)	1 piece	10	1.7
Iced (Sunshine)	1 piece	26	3.7

Food and Description	Measure or Quantity	Calories	Carbo-hydrates (grams)
Butterscotch Fudgies *(Tastykake)*	1 pkg. (1¾ oz.)	251	35.0
Capri *(Pepperidge Farm)*	1 piece	82	9.7
Cardiff *(Pepperidge Farm)*	1 piece	18	2.5
Cherry Coolers *(Sunshine)*	1 piece	29	4.5
Chinese almond (Stella D'oro)	1 piece	178	21.5
Chocolate & chocolate-covered			
(USDA)	1 oz.	126	20.3
(Van de Kamp's)	1 piece	79	
Como *(Stella D'oro)*	1 piece	155	16.8
Creme *(Wise)*	1 piece	32	4.9
Peanut bars, Ideal *(Nabisco)*	1 piece	94	10.3
Pinwheels *(Nabisco)*	1 piece	139	29
Snaps *(Nabisco)*	1 piece	18	2.7
(Sunshine)	1 piece	14	2.4
Wafers, famous *(Nabisco)*	1 piece	28	4.7
Chocolate chip, home recipe, with enriched flour *(USDA)*	1 cookie	50	6
	1 oz.	146	17.0
Chocolate chip, Commercial (USDA)	1 cookie	50	7
	1 oz.	134	19.8
Chocolate chip *(Pepperidge Farm)*	1 piece	52	6.2
(Van de Kamp's)	1 piece	66	
Chips Ahoy *(Nabisco)*	3 cookies	160	22
Family favorites *(Nabisco)*	1 piece	33	4.5
Old fashioned *(Keebler)*	1 piece	80	11.0
Snaps *(Nabisco)*	1 piece	21	3.4
Chip-A-Roos *(Sunshine)*	11.6 gr. per biscuit	63	7.7
Choc-O-Chip *(Tastykake)*	4 pieces (1¾-oz. pkg.)	283	34.8
Chocolate chip coconut *(Sunshine)*	15.7 gr. per biscuit	80	9.7
Cinnamon, crisp *(Keebler)*	1 piece	17	2.7

Food and Description	Measure or Quantity	Calories	Carbohydrates (grams)
Spice, vanilla sandwich, Crinkles (Nabisco)	6 pieces (1-5/8-oz. pkg.)	228	33.4
Sugar (Pepperidge Farm)	1 piece	52	7.0
Toast (Sunshine)	1 piece	13	2.3
Coconut bar (USDA)	1 oz.	140	18.1
(Nabisco)	1 piece	45	6.3
(Sunshine)	1 piece	47	6.2
Coconut, Family Favorites (Nabisco)	1 piece	16	2.2
Chocolate chip (Nabisco)	1 piece	77	9.0
Chocolate drop (Keebler)	1 piece	75	8.5
Coconut Kiss (Tastykake)	4 pieces (1¾-oz. pkg.)	318	33.2
Jumble (Drake's)	1 piece	70	10.6
Commodore (Keebler)	1 piece	65	10.1
Como Delight (Stella D'oro)	1 piece	153	18.3
Cowboys & Indians (Nabisco)	1 piece	10	1.8
Cream Lunch (Sunshine)	1 piece	45	7.3
Cream Wafer Stick (Dutch Twin)	1 piece	36	5.9
(Nabisco)	1 piece	50	5.9
Cup Custard, Chocolate (Sunshine)	1 piece	70	9.3
Vanilla (Sunshine)	1 piece	71	9.3
Devil's Food Cake (Nab)	2 pieces (1¼-oz. pkg.)	135	26.8
(Nabisco)	1 piece	49	9.8
Dixie Vanilla (Sunshine)	1 piece	60	13.1
Dresden (Pepperidge Farm)	1 piece	83	10.0
Dutch Girl (Van de Kamp's)	1 piece	53	
Egg Jumbo (Stella D'oro)	1 piece	40	7.6
Fig bars, Commercial (USDA)	1 cookie	50	11
	1 oz.	101	21.4
(Keebler)	1 piece	71	14.4
(Sunshine)	1 piece	45	9.2

C
D

Food and Description	Measure or Quantity	Calories	Carbo-hydrates (grams)
Fig Newtons (Nab)	1 piece (1-oz. pkg.)	104	20.2
	2 pieces (2-oz. pkg.)	208	40.4
Fig Newtons (Nabisco)	2 cakes	110	23
Fortune (Chun King)	1 piece	31	4.6
Fruit, Iced (Nabisco)	1 piece	71	13.5
Fudge (Sunshine)	1 piece	72	9.4
Chip (Pepperidge Farm)	1 piece	51	6.7
Fudge Stripes (Keebler)	1 piece	57	7.5
Gingersnap (USDA)	1 oz.	119	22.6
(Keebler)	1 piece	24	4.3
Old fashion (Nabisco)	1 piece	29	5.4
(Sunshine)	1 piece	24	4.4
ZuZu (Nabisco)	1 piece	16	3.1
Golden Bars (Stella D'oro)	1 piece	123	16.0
Golden Fruit (Sunshine)	18.5 gr. per biscuit	61	14.4
Hermit bar, Frosted (Tastykake)	1 pkg. (2 oz.)	321	60.8
Home Plate (Keebler)	1 piece	58	9.9
Hostess With the Mostest (Stella D'oro)	1 piece	39	5.2
Hydrox, Regular or mint (Sunshine)	1 piece	48	7.1
Vanilla (Sunshine)	10.1 gr. per biscuit	50	7.1
Jan Hagel (Keebler)	1 piece	44	6.7
Keebies (Keebler)	1 piece	51	7.1
Ladyfingers (USDA)	.4-oz. lady-finger	40	7.1
Lemon (Sunshine)	15.1 gr. per biscuit	76	9.8
Jumble rings (Nabisco)	1 piece	68	11.0
Lemon Coolers (Sunshine)	1 piece	29	4.5
Lemon Nut Crunch (Pepperidge Farm)	1 piece	57	6.4
Lemon Snaps (Nabisco)	1 piece	17	3.1

Food and Description	Measure or Quantity	Calories	Carbohydrates (grams)
Lido (Pepperidge Farm)	1 piece	91	10.0
Lisbon (Pepperidge Farm)	1 piece	28	3.3
Macaroon (USDA)	1 oz.	116	20.5
Almond (Tastykake)	2 pieces (2-oz. pkg.)	336	35.0
Coconut, Bake Shop (Nabisco)	1 piece	87	12.1
Coconut (Van de Kamp's)	1 piece	89	
Sandwich (Nabisco)	1 piece	71	9.5
Mallopuffs (Sunshine)	16.5 gr. per biscuit	63	12.2
Margherite, Chocolate (Stella D'oro)	1 piece	73	10.6
Vanilla (Stella D'oro)	1 piece	73	10.5
Marquisette (Pepperidge Farm)	1 piece	45	5.0
Marshmallow (USDA)	1 oz.	116	20.5
Fancy Crests (Nabisco)	1 piece	53	10.4
Mallowmars (Nabisco)	1 piece	60	8.7
Minarets (Nabisco)	1 piece	46	5.7
Puffs (Nabisco)	1 piece	94	12.8
Sandwich (Nabisco)	1 piece	32	5.7
Twirls (Nabisco)	1 piece	133	21.9
Milano (Pepperidge Farm)	1 piece	62	7.2
Mint (Pepperidge Farm)	1 piece	76	8.4
Mint sandwich, Mystic (Nabisco)	1 piece	88	10.6
Molasses (USDA)	1 oz.	120	21.5
Molasses & Spice (Sunshine)	1 piece	67	11.9
Naples (Pepperidge Farm)	1 piece	33	3.7
Nassau (Pepperidge Farm)	1 piece	83	9.2
Oatmeal (Nabisco)	1 piece	82	12.3
(Sunshine)	12.6 gr. per biscuit	58	1.5
(Van de Kamp's)	1 piece	59	
Family Favorites (Nabisco)	1 piece	24	3.8
Iced oatmeal (Sunshine)	15.3 gr. per biscuit	69	11.6
Irish (Pepperidge Farm)	1 piece	50	7.1
Old fashioned (Keebler)	1 piece	79	11.7
Peanut butter (Sunshine)	1 piece	79	10.5
Raisin (USDA)	1 oz.	128	20.8

C
D

Food and Description	Measure or Quantity	Calories	Carbohydrates (grams)
Raisin, Bake Shop (Nabisco)	1 piece	77	11.5
Raisin (Pepperidge Farm)	1 piece	55	7.5
Raisin bar (Tastykake)	1 pkg. (2¼ oz.)	298	47.6
Whole wheat (Drake's)	1 piece	75	11.4
Old Country Treats (Stella D'oro)	1 piece	64	7.1
Orleans (Pepperidge Farm)	1 piece	30	3.5
Peach-apricot pastry (Stella D'oro)	1 piece	99	15.0
Peanut & peanut butter (USDA)	1 oz.	134	19.0
Bars, cocoa covered, Crowns (Nabisco)	1 piece	92	10.0
Caramel logs, Heydays (Nabisco)	1 piece	122	13.4
Creme patties (Nab)	3 pieces (½-oz. pkg.)	74	8.4
Creme patties (Nab)	6 pieces (1-oz. pkg.)	148	16.8
Creme patties (Nabisco)	1 piece	34	3.9
Creme patties, cocoa covered, Fancy (Nabisco)	1 piece	60	6.4
Patties (Sunshine)	1 piece	33	4.2
Sandwich, Nutter Butter (Nabisco)	1 piece	69	9.2
Pecan Sandies (Keebler)	1 piece	85	9.2
Penguins (Keebler)	1 piece	111	14.0
Pfefferneuse, Spice drop (Stella D'oro)	1 piece	40	
Pirouette, Chocolate laced (Pepperidge Farm)	1 piece	38	4.5
Lemon or original (Pepperidge Farm)	1 piece	37	4.4
Pitter Patter (Keebler)	1 piece	84	10.9
Pizzelle, Carolines (Stella D'oro)	1 piece	49	6.7
Raisin (USDA)	1 oz.	107	22.9
Fruit Biscuit (Nabisco)	1 piece	58	12.3

Food and Description	Measure or Quantity	Calories	Carbohydrates (grams)
Rich'n Chips (Keebler)	1 piece	73	8.9
Rochelle (Pepperidge Farm)	1 piece	81	9.6
Sandwich, creme (USDA)	1 oz.	140	19.6
Chocolate or vanilla, Commercial (USDA)	1 cookie	50	7
Assorted, Cookie Break (Nabisco)	1 piece	52	7.0
Cameo (Nabisco)	1 piece	68	10.5
Chocolate chip (Nabisco)	1 piece	73	9.1
Chocolate fudge (Keebler)	1 piece	99	13.0
Chocolate, Cookie Break (Nabisco)	1 piece	53	7.1
Orbit (Sunshine)	1 piece	51	7.0
Oreo (Nab)	4 pieces (1-oz. pkg.)	140	20.1
Oreo (Nab)	6 pieces (1-5/8-oz. pkg.)	228	32.7
Oreo (Nab)	6 pieces (2-1/8-oz. pkg.)	298	32.7
Oreo chocolate sandwich Cookies (Nabisco)	3 cookies	150	22
Oreo & Swiss (Nab)	6 pieces (1-5/8-oz. pkg.)	230	31.4
Oreo & Swiss (Nab)	6 pieces (2¼-oz. pkg.)	319	43.6
Oreo & Swiss, Assortment (Nabisco)	1 piece	51	7.0
Pride (Nabisco)	1 piece	55	7.3
Social Tea (Nabisco)	1 piece	51	7.2
Swiss (Nabisco)	4 pieces (1-oz. pkg.)	144	18.2
Swiss (Nab)	6 pieces (1¾-oz. pkg.)	252	31.9

Food and Description	Measure or Quantity	Calories	Carbohydrates (grams)
Swiss (Nabisco)	1 piece	52	6.6
Vanilla (Keebler)	1 piece	82	11.1
Vanilla (Nabisco)	1 piece	52	7.0
Vienna Finger sandwich (Sunshine)	14.8 gr. per biscuit	71	10.5
Sesame, Regina (Stella D'oro)	1 piece	51	6.9
Shortbread (USDA)	1 oz.	141	18.5
Dandy (Nabisco)	1 piece	46	7.7
(Pepperidge Farm)	1 piece	72	8.3
Cherry nut (Van de Kamp's)	1 piece	59	
Lorna Doone (Nab)	4 pieces (1-oz. pkg.)	138	19.0
Lorna Doone (Nab)	6 pieces (1½-oz. pkg.)	207	28.5
Lorna Doone Shortbread (Nabisco)	4 cookies	160	19
Pecan (Nabisco)	1 piece	80	9.0
Scotties (Sunshine)	1 piece	39	5.0
Striped (Nabisco)	1 piece	50	6.8
Vanilla (Tastykake)	6 pieces (2¼-oz. pkg.)	352	43.8
Social Tea Biscuit (Nabisco)	6 biscuits	120	21
Spiced wafers (Nabisco)	1 piece	41	7.4
Sprinkles (Sunshine)	1 piece	57	11.4
Sugar cookie (Pepperidge Farm)	1 piece	51	7.0
(Sunshine)	17.5 gr. per biscuit	86	11.9
(Van de Kamp's)	1 piece	79	
Brown, Family Favorite (Nabisco)	1 piece	25	3.0
Brown (Pepperidge Farm)	1 piece	48	6.9
Old fashioned (Keebler)	1 piece	78	12.4
Rings (Nabisco)	1 piece	69	10.7
Sugar wafer (USDA)	1 oz.	137	20.8
(Sunshine)	8.9 gr. per biscuit	43	6.6

Food and Description	Measure or Quantity	Calories	Carbohydrates (grams)
Assorted *(Dutch Twin)*	1 piece	34	4.7
Biscos *(Nab)*	3 pieces (7/8-oz. pkg.)	128	17.5
Sugar wafers, Biscos			
(Nabisco)	8 wafers	150	20
Krisp Kreme *(Keebler)*	1 piece	31	3.7
Lemon *(Sunshine)*	1 piece	44	6.5
Swedish Kreme *(Keebler)*	1 piece	31	3.7
Tahiti *(Pepperidge Farm)*	1 piece	84	8.6
Toy cookies *(Sunshine)*	2.8 gr. per biscuit	13	2.1
Vanilla creme *(Wise)*	1 piece	33	5.0
Vanilla snap *(Nabisco)*	1 piece	13	2.3
Vanilla wafer *(USDA)*	1 oz.	131	21.1
(Keebler)	1 piece	18	2.9
Nilla *(Nabisco)*	7 wafers	130	21
Vanilla wafers, small			
(Sunshine)	3.1 gr. per wafer	15	2.2
Venice *(Pepperidge Farm)*	1 piece	57	6.3
Waffle creme *(Dutch Twin)*	1 piece	44	6.1
Biscos *(Nabisco)*	1 piece	42	6.0
Yum Yums *(Sunshine)*	1 piece	83	10.4

COOKIES — DIETETIC

Food and Description	Measure or Quantity	Calories	Carbohydrates (grams)
Almond chocolate wafer *(Estee)*	1 piece	27	2.6
Angel puffs *(Stella D'oro)*	1 piece	17	1.5
Apple pastry *(Stella D'oro)*	1 piece	94	13.6
Assorted *(Estee)*	1 piece	31	4.8
Assorted filled wafers *(Estee)*	1 piece	25	3.2
Banana wafers *(Estee)*	1 piece	123	10.4
Beljuin Treats *(Estee)*	1 piece	32	3.2
Chocolate chip *(Estee)*	1 piece	32	3.6
Chocolate, Holland-filled wafer (Estee)	1 piece	22	2.0
Chocolate & vanilla wafer (Estee)	1 piece	27	3.2

Food and Description	Measure or Quantity	Calories	Carbohydrates (grams)
Fig pastry (Stella D'oro)	1 piece	100	15.5
Fruit flavored wafer (Estee)	1 piece	22	2.0
Have-A-Heart (Stella D'oro)	1 piece	97	11.3
Holland bittersweet wafer (Estee)	1 piece	127	10.4
Holland milk chocolate wafer (Estee)	1 piece	127	10.4
Kichel (Stella D'oro)	1 piece	8	.7
Mint, chocolate (Estee)	1 piece	4	1.0
Mint, fruit flavors (Estee)	1 piece	4	1.0
Monties (Estee)	1 piece	38	2.5
Oatmeal raisin (Estee)	1 piece	36	4.4
Pastry stick (Estee)	1 piece	40	4.3
Peach-apricot pastry (Stella D'oro)	1 piece	104	15.2
Prune pastry (Stella D'oro)	1 piece	92	14.3
Royal Nuggets (Stella D'oro)	1 piece	2	.1
Sandwich, chocolate (Estee)	1 piece	42	4.6
Sandwich, Duplex (Estee)	1 piece	42	4.8
Sandwich, Lemon (Estee)	1 piece	69	7.8
Vanilla filled wafer (Estee)	1 piece	25	3.2
Vanilla Holland filled wafer (Estee)	1 piece	22	2.0
Vanilla & strawberry wafer (Estee)	1 piece	25	3.2
Wafer cake (Estee)	1 piece	44	4.5
COOKIE MIXES			
Butterscotch nut (Pillsbury)**	3 cookies	120	16
Chocolate chip (Pillsbury)**	3 cookies	130	19
Peanut butter (Pillsbury)**	3 cookies	130	15
Sugar cookie (Pillsbury)**	3 cookies	130	19
Oatmeal chocolate chip (Pillsbury)**	3 cookies	130	18
Oatmeal raisin (Pillsbury)**	3 cookies	140	20
Brownies (USDA)	1 brownie	85	13
(Duncan Hines)	1 brownie	150	20

** Baked from refrigerated cookie dough.

100

Food and Description	Measure or Quantity	Calories	Carbohydrates (grams)
Fudge brownies (Pillsbury)	2, 1½-in. square	120	19
Lemon (Nestle's)	1 oz.	132	20.1
Plain, dry *(USDA)	1 oz.	140	18.9
Sugar (Nestle's)	1 oz.	132	20.1
Toll House (Nestle's)	1 oz.	132	20.1
Toll House, with morsels, prepared with egg *(Nestle's)	1 piece (.4 oz.)	52	7.2

CRACKERS, PUFFS, CHIPS

Food and Description	Measure or Quantity	Calories	Carbohydrates (grams)
Arrowroot biscuit (Nabisco)	1 piece	22	3.5
Bacon flavored thins (Nabisco)	1 piece	11	1.2
Bacon toast (Keebler)	1 piece	15	2.0
Bakon Tasters (Old London)	½-oz. bag	62	8.8
Bakon Delites, Regular (Wise)	½-oz. bag	72	0
Barbecue flavor (Wise)	½-oz. bag	70	.3
Bugles (General Mills)	15 pieces	81	7.5
Butter thins (Nabisco)	1 piece	15	2.4
Cheese 'n Bacon Sandwich (Nab)	6 pieces (1¼-oz. pkg.)	179	18.9
Cheese 'n Cracker (Kraft)	4 crackers & ¾-oz. cheese	138	.7
Cheese Nips (Nab)	24 pieces (7/8-oz. pkg.)	114	16.5
(Nabisco)	1 piece (1 gram)	5	.7
Cheese & Peanut Butter Sandwich, Squares (Nab)	6 pieces (1½-oz. pkg.)	208	22.1
Squares (Nab)	4 pieces (1-oz. pkg.)	139	14.7

*Prepared as package directs.

101

Food and Description	Measure or Quantity	Calories	Carbohydrates (grams)
Variety pack (Nab)	6 pieces (1½-oz. pkg.)	209	22.7
Cheese on Rye Sandwich (Nab)	6 pieces (1¼-oz. pkg.)	191	17.6
Cheese Pixies (Wise)	1-oz. bag	163	13.4
Chee Tos, Cheese-flavored puffs.	1 oz.	156	15.2
Cheez Doodles (Old London)	1-1/8-oz. bag	170	18.5
Cheez-Its (Sunshine)	1 piece (1 gram)	6	.6
Chicken in a Biskit (Nabisco)	1 piece (2 grams)	10	1.2
Chippers (Nabisco)	1 piece (3 grams)	14	1.8
Club crackers (Keebler)	1 piece (3 grams)	15	2.0
Corn chips (Fritos)	1 oz.	161	15.3
(Old London)	1¾-oz. bag	263	27.3
(Wise)	1¾-oz. bag	276	27.6
Taco (Old London)	1½-oz. bag	167	23.8
Corn Diggers (Nabisco)	1 piece	4	.5
Cracker Crumbs, Graham (Keebler)	3 oz.	368	64.1
Graham (Nabisco)	1½ cups (4.6 oz. or 9 in. pie shell)	563	100.3
Graham (Sunshine)	3 oz.	357	66.2
Graham (USDA)	1 cup (3 oz.)	330	63.0
Cracker Meal (Sunshine)	3 oz.	340	71.2
(USDA)	3 oz.	373	60.0
Fine, medium or coarse (Keebler)	3 oz.	316	68.5

Food and Description	Measure or Quantity	Calories	Carbohydrates (grams)
Salted (Nabisco)	1 cup (3 oz.)	309	65.7
Unsalted (Nabisco)	1 cup (3 oz.)	319	67.9
Croutettes (Kellogg's)	7-oz. dry mix	70	15
Dipsy Doodles (Old London)	1¾-oz. bag	276	26.4
Doo Dads (Nabisco)	1 piece	2	.3
Escort crackers (Nabisco)	7 crackers	150	19
Flings, Cheese flavored curls (Nabisco)	1 piece	11	.6
Swiss 'n Ham (Nabisco)	1 piece	10	.8
Goldfish (Pepperidge Farm)			
Cheddar cheese	10 pieces	28	3.3
Lightly salted	10 pieces	28	3.6
Parmesan cheese	10 pieces	29	3.4
Pizza	10 pieces	29	3.6
Pretzel	10 pieces	29	5.0
Onion	10 pieces	28	3.6
Sesame garlic	10 pieces	29	3.5
Graham crackers (USDA)	2½-in. sq.	27	5.1
2½-in square (USDA)	4 crackers	110	21
Honey Maid graham crackers (Nabisco)	4 crackers	120	22
Chocolate or cocoa-covered, Deluxe (Keebler)	1 piece	42	5.6
Chocolate or cocoa-covered, Pantry (Nabisco)	1 piece	62	8.5
Sugar-honey coated (USDA)	1 oz.	117	21.7
Hi-Ho crackers (Sunshine)	1 piece	18	2.1
Krispy crackers (Sunshine)	2.7 gr. per biscuit	11	2
Meal Mates (Nabisco)	1 piece	19	3.4
Melba Toast, Garlic (Keebler)	1 piece	9	1.5
Garlic, round (Old London)	1 piece	8	1.4
Onion (Keebler)	1 piece	9	1.5
Onion, round (Old London)	1 piece	8	1.4
Plain (Keebler)	1 piece	9	1.5
Pumpernickel (Old London)	1 piece	15	3.0

C
D

Food and Description	Measure or Quantity	Calories	Carbohydrates (grams)
Rye (Old London)	1 piece	14	3.1
Rye, unsalted (Old London)	1 piece	15	3.3
Sesame (Keebler)	1 piece	11	1.4
Sesame, rounds (Old London)	1 piece	9	1.2
Wheat (Old London)	1 piece	15	3.1
Wheat, unsalted (Old London)	1 piece	15	3.2
White (Keebler)	1 piece	16	3.3
White (Old London)	1 piece	15	3.1
White, unsalted (Old London)	1 piece	15	3.2
Milk lunch cracker, Royal Lunch (Nabisco)	1 piece	55	7.9
Munchos, Onion flavored	1 oz.	148	15.8
OTC (Original Trenton Cracker)	1 cracker	23	4.4
Oyster, cracker (USDA)	10 pieces	44	7.1
Mini cracker (Sunshine)	.8 gr. per biscuit	3	.6
Oysterettes (Nabisco)	1 piece	3	.6
Peanut butter sandwich, Cheese crackers (Wise)	1 piece	30	3.4
Malted milk crackers (Nab)	6 pieces (1-3/8-oz. pkg.)	189	22.1
Pizza Spins (General Mills)	32 pieces	72	8.0
Potato crisps (General Mills)	16 pieces	78	7.5
Popcorn, popped, sugar coated (USDA)	1 cup	135	30
Popped with oil & salt (USDA)	1 cup	40	5
Popped, plain large kernel (USDA)	1 cup	25	5
Pop-tarts, cherry (Kellogg's)	1 pastry	210	35
Cherry, frosted (Kellogg's)	1 pastry	210	36
Pretzels, Dutch twisted (USDA)	1 pretzel	60	12
Thin, twisted (USDA)	1 pretzel	25	5
Veri-thin (Mister Salty, Nabisco)	5 pretzels	100	20
Pretzel sticks, 3-1/8 in. (USDA)	5 sticks	10	2
Ritz cracker, plain (Nabisco)	1 piece	16	2.1
Cheese flavored (Nabisco)	9 crackers	150	18

Food and Description	Measure or Quantity	Calories	Carbohydrates (grams)
Ry-Krisp crackers, Seasoned.	1 whole cracker	27	4.5
Traditional.	1 whole cracker	23	4.8
Rye thins (Pepperidge Farm)	1 piece	10	2.0
Saltines (USDA)	4 crackers	50	8
Flavor-Kist, Any kind	1 piece	12	2.2
Krispy, salted tops (Sunshine)	1 piece	11	2.0
Krispy, unsalted tops (Sunshine)	1 piece	12	2.1
Premium (Nabisco)	10 crackers	120	20
Zesta (Keebler)	1 piece	12	2.0
Sea Toast, crackers (Keebler)	1 piece	62	11.1
Sesame cracker, Buttery flavor (Nabisco)	1 piece	16	1.9
Wafer, Meal Mates (Nabisco)	1 piece	21	3.2
Shapies, Dip delights (Nabisco)	1 piece (2 grams)	9	.8
Shells (Nabisco)	1 piece (2 grams)	10	.9
Sip 'N Chips (Nabisco)	1 piece	9	1.0
Sociables, crackers (Nabisco)	1 piece	10	1.3
Soda cracker, Premium, unsalted tops (Nabisco)	1 piece	12	2.0
Soda crackers (Sunshine)	4.5 gr. per biscuit	20	3.3
Thins, Dietetic (Estee)	1 piece	6	.9
Toast (Keebler)	1 piece (3 grams)	16	1.9
Toasty, crackers (Austin's)	1 piece	37	0
Tortilla chips (Old London)	1½-oz. bag	207	27.8
(Wonder)	1 oz.	148	17.2
Doritos (Frito-Lay)	1 oz.	140	18.7
Town House Crackers	1 piece	18	2.0
Triangle Thins (Nabisco)	1 piece	8	1.1
Triscuit, wafers (Nabisco)	7 wafers	140	21
Twigs, sesame & cheese, crackers (Nabisco)	1 piece	14	1.6

C
D

Food and Description	Measure or Quantity	Calories	Carbohydrates (grams)
Uneeda Biscuit, unsalted tops (Nabisco)	1 piece	22	3.7
Wafer-ets, crackers, Rice, salted (Hol-Grain)	1 piece	12	2.5
Rice, unsalted (Hol-Grain)	1 piece	12	2.5
Wheat, salted (Hol-Grain)	1 piece	7	1.4
Wheat, unsalted (Hol-Grain)	1 piece	7	1.4
Waldorf, crackers, Low salt (Keebler)	1 piece	14	2.4
Waverly, Wafer (Nabisco)	1 piece	18	2.6
Wheat chips (General Mills)	12 pieces	73	7.8
Wheat thins (Nabisco)	16 crackers	140	19
Wheat toast (Keebler)	1 cracker	16	2.0
Whistles (General Mills)	17 chips	71	8.0
White thins (Pepperidge Farm)	1 cracker	12	2.0
Whole-wheat crackers, (USDA)	1 oz.	114	19.3
Natural, crackers (Froumine)	1 piece (.4 oz.)	46	7.5

DESSERTS

Food and Description	Measure or Quantity	Calories	Carbohydrates (grams)
Apple Brown Betty, Home Recipe (USDA)	1 cup	347	68.3
Charlotte Russe, With ladyfingers, whipped cream filling, Home recipe (USDA)	4 oz.	324	38.0
Eclair, Home recipe with custard filling & chocolate icing (USDA)	1 4oz.	271	26.3
Golden Egg Custard, Mix (Jello)	½ cup	170	6
Milk desserts, Custard, baked (USDA)	1 cup	305	24
Pie Filling, Lemon (Royal)	1 sector	220	39.8
Puddings, Banana Pudding, canned (Del Monte)	5-oz. container	187	31.7
Banana Pudding & Pie Mix, Instant *(Jello)	½ cup (5.3 oz.)	178	30.5
Instant *(Royal)	½ cup (5.1 oz.)	177	30.5

*Prepared as package directs.

Food and Description	Measure or Quantity	Calories	Carbo-hydrates (grams)
Regular *(Jello)	½ cup (5.2 oz.)	173	29.3
Regular *(My-T-Fine)	½ cup (5 oz.)	175	32.6
Regular *(Royal)	½ cup (5.1 oz.)	168	27.6
Bavarian Pie or Pudding Mix, Cream *(My-T-Fine)	½ cup (5 oz.)	175	32.5
Custard *(Rice-A-Roni)	4 oz.	143	24.6
Butterscotch Pudding or Pie Mix, Sweetened, Regular			
*(My-T-Fine)	½ cup	175	32.5
*(Royal)	½ cup	191	31.8
Sweetened, Instant *(Jello)	½ cup	178	30.5
Sweetened, Instant *(Royal)	½ cup	177	29.0
Low calorie *(D-Zerta)	½ cup	107	4.8
Chocolate pudding, Home recipe with starch base (USDA)	1 cup	385	67
Regular (Royal)	½ cup	190	31.7
Instant (Royal)	½ cup	190	31.8
Pudding cup (Del Monte)	5 oz.	190	31
Snack pack (Hunt)	5 oz.	180	24
Chocolate Pudding & Pie Filling (Jello)	½ cup	170	28
Instant (Jello)	½ cup	190	34
Lemon Pudding & Pie Filling (Jello)	1/6 of 9-in. pie	180	38
Instant (Jello)	½ cup	180	31
Pudding mix, dry form, 4-oz. pkg. (USDA)	1 pkg.	410	103
Vanilla pudding, Home recipe with starch base (USDA)	1 cup	285	41
Instant (Royal)	½ cup	190	28.8
Regular (Royal)	½ cup	160	26.4
Pudding cup (Del Monte)	5 oz.	190	32
Snack pack (Hunt)	5 oz.	190	26

* Prepared as pkg. directs.

Food and Description	Measure or Quantity	Calories	Carbohydrates (grams)
Vanilla Pudding & Pie Filling			
(Jello)	½ cup	170	27
Instant (Jello)	½ cup	180	31
Low Calorie (D-Zerta)	½ cup	70	13
Sherbert (USDA)	1 cup	260	59
Tapioca dessert, Apple (USDA)	1 cup	295	74
Tapioca, dry, quick cooking (USDA)	1 cup	535	131
Tapioca pudding, Chocolate (Jello)	½ cup	170	28
Snack pack (Hunt)	5 oz.	130	23
Vanilla (Jello)	½ cup	170	28
EGGS			
Boiled (USDA)	1 large egg	81	.4
Egg Beaters, Cholesterol free egg substitute (Fleischmann)	¼ cup	90	3
Fried in butter (USDA)	1 large egg	99	.1
Large, 24 oz. per dozen, Raw cook in shell, or with nothing added, Whole, without shell (USDA)	1 egg	80	Trace
Omelet, mixed with milk & cooked in fat (USDA)	1 large egg	107	1.5
Poached (USDA)	1 large egg	78	.4
Raw, Whole (USDA)	1 cup	409	2.3
Whole, Small (USDA)	1 egg	60	.3
Whole, Medium (USDA)	1 egg	71	.4
Whole, Large (USDA)	1 egg	81	.4
Whole, Extra Large (USDA)	1 egg	94	.5
Whole, Jumbo (USDA)	1 egg	105	.6
Scrambled eggs and link sausage, With coffee cake, frozen breakfast (Swanson)	1 complete breakfast	460	22
Scrambled, With milk & fat (USDA)	1 egg	110	1
White of egg (USDA)	1 white	15	Trace

*Prepared as package directs.

Food and Description	Measure or Quantity	Calories	Carbohydrates (grams)
Yolks of egg (USDA)	1 yolk	60	Trace
FATS, OILS			
Butter, Regular, 4 sticks per lb. (USDA)	1 tbsp.	100	Trace
Pat, 1-in. sq., 1/3 in. high (USDA)	1 pat	35	Trace
Lightly salted (Breakstone–Sugar Creek Foods)	1 pat	100	.5
Sweet, unsalted (Breakstone–Sugar Creek Foods)	1 pat	100	.6
Whipped, approx. 1/8 stick (USDA)	1 tbsp.	65	Trace
Whipped, pat 1¼ in. sq., 1/3 in. high (USDA)	1 pat	25	Trace
Whipped, lightly salted (Breakstone–Sugar Creek Foods)	1 pat	65	.5
Whipped, sweet (Breakstone–Sugar Creek Foods)	1 pat	65	.6
Whipped (Sealtest)	1 tbsp.	68	.1
Margarine (Blue Bonnet)	1 tbsp.	100	.10
(Nucoa)	1 tbsp.	100	0
Regular (Fleischmann's)	1 tbsp.	100	.10
Regular (Parkay)	1 tbsp.	101	.1
Regular (USDA)	1 tbsp.	100	Trace
Corn Oil (Miracle)	1 tbsp.	67	<.1
Corn oil deluxe (Parkay)	1 tbsp.	101	.1
Danish flavor (Borden)	1 tbsp.	101	<.1
Imitation, diet (Fleischmann's)	1 tbsp.	50	.1
(Imperial)	1 tbsp.	48	0
(Mazola)	1 tbsp.	50	0
(Mazola)	1 cup	804	0
(Parkay)	1 tbsp.	55	0
Safflower oil, soft (Parkay)	1 tbsp.	95	.1
Soft (Blue Bonnet)	1 tbsp.	100	.10
(Fleischmann's)	1 tbsp.	100	.10
(Mazola)	1 tbsp.	100	0

Food and Description	Measure or Quantity	Calories	Carbo-hydrates (grams)
(USDA)	1 tbsp.	100	Trace
Soft, polyunsaturated *(Nucoa)*	1 tbsp.	90	0
Stick *(Promise)*	1 tbsp.	102	.1
Unsalted *(Fleischmann's)*	1 tbsp.	100	.10
(Mazola)	1 tbsp.	100	0
Whipped *(Blue Bonnet)*	1 tbsp.	70	.06
(Imperial)	1 tbsp.	68	<.1
Whipped, Cup *(Parkay)*	1 tbsp.	67	<.1
Cooking Fats, Crisco *(Proctor & Gamble)*	1 tbsp.	110	0
Fluffo *(Proctor & Gamble)*	1 tbsp.	110	0
Lard *(USDA)*	1 tbsp.	115	0
Vegetable fats *(USDA)*	1 tbsp.	110	0
Salad or Cooking Oils, Corn Oil *(Mazola)*	1 tbsp.	120	0
Corn oil *(USDA)*	1 tbsp.	125	0
Cottonseed Oil *(USDA)*	1 tbsp.	125	0
Crisco Oil *(Proctor & Gamble)*	1 tbsp.	120	0
Olive Oil *(USDA)*	1 tbsp.	125	0
Peanut Oil *(USDA)*	1 tbsp.	125	0
Safflower Oil *(USDA)*	1 tbsp.	125	0
Soybean Oil *(USDA)*	1 tbsp.	125	0
Soybean & Cottonseed Oil *(Wesson)*	1 tbsp.	120	0

FISH

Food and Description	Measure or Quantity	Calories	Carbo-hydrates (grams)
Barracuda, raw, meat only *(USDA)*	4 oz.	128	0
Bass, Black sea, raw, whole *(USDA)*	1 lb. (weighed whole)	165	0
Blacksea, Baked, Home recipe, stuffed with bacon, butter, onion, celery & bread cubes *(USDA)*	4 oz.	294	12.9

Food and Description	Measure or Quantity	Calories	Carbohydrates (grams)
Black sea, whole, Smallmouth & largemouth, raw *(USDA)*	1 lb. (weighed whole)	146	0
Black sea, Smallmouth & largemouth, meat only *(USDA)*	4 oz.	118	0
Striped, raw, whole *(USDA)*	1 lb. (weighed whole)	205	0
Striped, raw, meat only *(USDA)*	4 oz.	119	0
Striped, oven-fried, made with milk, breadcrumbs & butter *(USDA)*	4 oz.	222	7.6
White, raw, whole *(USDA)*	1 lb. (weighed whole)	173	0
White, raw, meat only *(USDA)*	4 oz.	111	0
Bluefish, Baked with table fat *(USDA)*	3 oz.	135	0
Carp, raw, whole *(USDA)*	1 lb. (weighed whole)	156	0
Meat only *(USDA)*	4 oz.	130	0
Caviar, Sturgeon, Pressed.	1 oz.	90	1.4
Whole eggs.	1 oz.	74	.9
Whole eggs.	1 tbsp. (.6 oz.)	42	.5
Clams, raw, meat only *(USDA)*	3 oz.	65	2
Raw, all kinds, meat & liquid *(USDA)*	4 oz.	60	2.8
Raw, all kinds, meat only *(USDA)*	4 med. clams (3 oz.)	65	1.7

Food and Description	Measure or Quantity	Calories	Carbo-hydrates (grams)
Raw, soft, meat & liquid (USDA)	1 lb. (weighed in shell)	142	5.3
Clams, canned, solids & liquid (USDA)	3 oz.	45	2
Canned, solids & liquid, chopped & minced (Doxsee)	4 oz.	59	3.2
Canned, chopped, meat only (Doxsee)	4 oz.	111	2.1
Canned, chopped (Snow)	4 oz.	68	2.4
Crab, all species, fresh, steamed, whole (USDA)	1 lb. (weighed in shell)	202	1.1
All species, fresh, steamed, Meat only (USDA)	1 cup	116	.6
Canned Crabmeat (USDA)	3 oz.	85	1
Canned, Alaska King (Del Monte)	7½-oz. can	202	3.6
Canned, solids & liquid, Fancy, King Crab (Icy Point)	7½-oz. can	215	2.3
(Pillar Rock)	7½-oz. can	215	2.3
Deviled, Home recipe, made with bread cubes, butter, parsley, eggs, lemon juice, catsup (USDA)	1 cup	451	31.9
Imperial, Home recipe, made with butter, flour, milk, onion, green pepper, eggs, Lemon juice (USDA)	1 cup	323	8.6
Croaker, Atlantic, raw, whole (USDA)	½ lb. (weighed whole)	148	0
Atlantic, Baked (USDA)	4 oz.	151	0
Eel, raw, meat only (USDA)	4 oz.	264	0
Smoked, meat only (USDA)	4 oz.	374	0
Fish cake (Beach Haven)	two	220	20
Gefilte Fish, 2-lb. jar			

Food and Description	Measure or Quantity	Calories	Carbohydrates (grams)
(Manischewitz)	1 piece (2.4 oz.)	64	2.5
1-lb. jar (Manischewitz)	1 piece (2.2 oz.)	60	2.3
4-piece can (Manischewitz)	1 piece (3.7 oz.)	100	3.9
Fish balls (Manischewitz)	1 piece (1.5 oz.)	40	1.6
Fishlets (Manischewitz)	1 piece (7 grams)	7	.3
Regular, ¼ of 1-lb. jar (Mother's)	1 piece (4 oz.)	55	3.5
Regular, 1/8 of 2-lb. jar (Mother's)	1 piece (4 oz.)	55	3.5
Whitefish & pike, 2-lb. jar (Manischewitz)	1 piece (1.7 oz.)	40	1.5
Whitefish & pike, 1-lb. jar (Manischewitz)	1 piece (1.5 oz.)	35	1.3
Whitefish & pike, Fishlets (Manischewitz)	1 piece (7 grams)	6	.2
Haddock, Breaded, fried (USDA)	3 oz.	140	5
Halibut, Atlantic & Pacific Raw, meat only (USDA)	4 oz.	113	0
California, raw, meat only (USDA)	4 oz.	110	0
Herring, Bismark, drained (Vita)	5-oz. jar	273	6.9
In cream sauce (Vita)	8-oz. jar	397	18.1
In wine sauce drained (Vita)	8-oz. jar	401	16.6
Tastee Bits, drained (Vita)	8-oz. jar	361	24.7
Smoked, Kippered (USDA)	4 oz. *	239	0
Lobster, Raw, whole (USDA)	1 lb. (weighed whole)	107	.6

Food and Description	Measure or Quantity	Calories	Carbo-hydrates (grams)
Raw, meat only (USDA)	4 oz.	103	.6
Cooked, meat only (USDA)	4 oz.	108	.3
Canned, meat only (USDA)	4 oz.	108	.3
Salad, home recipe (USDA)	4 oz.	125	2.6
Lobster Newburg, Home Recipe Made with butter, egg yolks, sherry & cream (USDA)	1 cup	485	12.8
Ocean Perch, Breaded, fried (USDA)	3 oz.	195	6
Oysters, Eastern, raw, meat only, 13-19 med. selects (USDA)	1 cup	160	8
Eastern, meat only (USDA)	4 oz.	75	3.9
Pacific & Western, meat only (USDA)	1 oz.	103	7.3
(USDA)	1 cup	218	15.4
Canned, solids & liquid (USDA)	4 oz.	86	5.6
Fried, dipped in egg, milk & bread crumbs (USDA)	4 oz.	271	21.1
Perch, raw, white, whole (USDA)	1 lb. (weighed whole)	193	0
White meat only (USDA)	4 oz.	134	0
Yellow, whole (USDA)	1 lb. (weighed whole)	161	0
Yellow, meat only (USDA)	4 oz.	103	0
Pike, Raw, Blue, whole (USDA)	1 lb. (weighed whole)	180	0
Raw, Blue, meat only (USDA)	4 oz.	102	0
Raw, Northern, whole (USDA)	1 lb. (weighed whole)	104	0
Raw, Northern, meat only (USDA)	4 oz.	100	0

Food and Description	Measure or Quantity	Calories	Carbohydrates (grams)
Raw, Walleye, whole(USDA)	1 lb. (weighed whole)	240	0
Raw, Walleye, meat only (USDA)	4 oz.	105	0
Rockfish, raw, meat only (USDA)	1 lb.	440	0
Oven-steamed with onion (USDA)	4 oz.	121	2.2
Roe, raw, carp, cod, haddock, Herring, pike or shad (USDA)	4 oz.	147	1.7
Salmon, raw, sturgeon turbot.	4 oz.	235	1.6
Baked or broiled with butter & lemon juice or vinegar, cod & shad (USDA)	4 oz.	143	2.2
Canned, cod, haddock or, herring, solids & liquid (USDA)	4 oz.	134	.3
Salmon, Atlantic, raw, whole (USDA)	1 lb. (weighed whole)	640	0
Atlantic, raw, Meat only (USDA)	4 oz.	246	0
Atlantic Canned, Solids & liquids, including bones (USDA)	4 oz.	230	0
Canned, solids & liquids (Pink Beauty)	7¾-oz. can	310	0
Chinook or King, raw, steak (USDA)	1 lb. (weighed with bones)	886	0
Chinook or King, meat only, raw (USDA)	4 oz.	252	0
Chinook or King, canned, solids & liquid, including bones (USDA)	4 oz.	238	0
Chum, canned, solids & liquid, including bones (USDA)	4 oz.	158	0
Coho, canned, solids & liquid, (USDA)	4 oz.	174	0

E
F

Food and Description	Measure or Quantity	Calories	Carbohydrates (grams)
Coho, canned, solids & liquid, Steak *(Icy Point)*	3¾-oz. can	162	0
Pink or Humpback, raw, steak *(USDA)*	1 lb. (weighed with bones)	475	0
Pink or humpback, raw meat only *(USDA)*	4 oz.	135	0
Pink or humpback, canned, solids & liquid *(USDA)*	4 oz.	160	0
Pink, canned *(Del Monte)*	7¾-oz.	310	0
Pink, canned, *(Icy Point)*	5¾-oz. can	310	0
Sockeye or Red, canned, solids & liquid, including bones *(USDA)*	4 oz.	194	0
(Del Monte)	7¾-oz. can	304	0
(Icy Point)	1-lb. can	775	0
(Pillar Rock)	1-lb. can	775	0
(Pillar Rock)	7¾-oz. can	376	0
(Pillar Rock)	3¾-oz. can	181	0
Unspecified kind of salmon, Baked or broiled with vegetable shortening *(USDA)*	4-oz. steak	218	0
(USDA)	5.1-oz. steak	264	0
Salmon Rice Loaf, Home recipe *(USDA)*	4 oz.	138	8.3
Salmon, Smoked *(USDA)*	4 oz.	200	0
Smoked Lox, drained *(Vita)*	4-oz. jar	136	.2
Smoked Nova, drained *(Vita)*	4-oz. can	221	1.0
Sardines, Atlantic, canned in oil, drained solids *(USDA)*	3 oz.	175	0
in mustard sauce *(Underwood)*	1 oz.	52	.6
In soy bean oil *(Underwood)*	1 oz.	62	.1
In tomato sauce *(Del Monte)*	7½ oz.	330	4
(Underwood)	1 oz.	45	1.2
Scallops, Raw, mussel only *(USDA)*	4 oz.	92	3.7
Steamed *(USDA)*	4 oz.	127	

Food and Description	Measure or Quantity	Calories	Carbohydrates (grams)
Shad, Raw, whole *(USDA)*	1 lb. (weighed whole)	370	0
Raw, Meat only *(USDA)*	4 oz.	193	0
Baked with table fat and bacon *(USDA)*	3 oz.	170	0
Cooked, Home recipe, Creole, Made with tomatoes, onion, green pepper, butter & flour *(USDA)*	4 oz.	172	1.8
Canned, Solids & liquid *(USDA)*	4 oz.	172	0
Sole, Raw, whole *(USDA)*	1 lb. (weighed whole)	118	0
Raw, Meat only *(USDA)*	4 oz.	90	0
Shrimp, Raw, whole *(USDA)*	1 lb. (weighed in shell)	285	4.7
Raw, Meat only *(USDA)*	4 oz.	103	1.7
Canned, meat *(USDA)*	3 oz.	100	1
Canned, Wet pack, solids & liquid *(USDA)*	4 oz.	91	.9
Canned, Cocktail, tiny, drained *(Icy Point)*	4½-oz. can	148	.8
Canned, tiny, drained *(Pillar Rock)*	4½-oz. can	148	.8
(Snow Mist)	4½-oz. can	148	.8
Cooked, french-fried, dipped in egg, bread crumbs & flour, or in batter *(USDA)*	4 oz.	255	11.3
Frozen, Raw, breaded, not more than 50% breading *(USDA)*	4 oz.	158	22.6
Frozen, Raw, breaded *(Chicken of The Sea)*	4 oz.	158	22.6
Smelt, Atlantic, jack & bay, Raw, whole *(USDA)*	1 lb. (weighed whole)	244	0

E F

Food and Description	Measure or Quantity	Calories	Carbohydrates (grams)
Raw, Meat only (USDA)	4 oz.	111	0
Canned, solids & liquid (USDA)	4 oz.	227	0
Snail, Raw (USDA)	4 oz.	102	2.3
Raw, Giant African (USDA)	4 oz.	83	5.0
Spot, Fillets, Raw (USDA)	1 lb.	993	0
Baked (USDA)	4 oz.	335	0
Sturgeon, Raw, section (USDA)	1 lb. (weighed with skin & bones)	362	0
Raw, Meat only (USDA)	4 oz.	107	0
Smoked (USDA)	4 oz.	169	0
Steamed (USDA)	4 oz.	181	0
Lake Trout, Raw, Drawn (USDA)	1 lb. (weighed with head, fins & bone)	282	0
Raw, Meat only (USDA)	4 oz.	191	0
Tuna, Raw, bluefin, meat only (USDA)	4 oz.	164	0
Raw, Yellowfin, meat only (USDA)	4 oz.	151	0
Canned in oil, drained solids (USDA)	3 oz.	170	0
Canned in oil, solids & liquid (USDA)	6½-oz. can	530	0
(Breast O'Chicken)	6½-oz. can	540	0
Chunk (Star-Kist)	3¼-oz. can	268	0
Chunk, light (Chicken of The Sea)	6-oz. can	405	0
(Del Monte)	1 cup (4.7 oz.)	346	0
Light, chunk in oil (Del Monte)	6½ oz.	450	0
Canned in oil, solids & liquid, solid (Star-Kist)	7-oz. can	577	0

Food and Description	Measure or Quantity	Calories	Carbohydrates (grams)
White albacore *(Del Monte)*	6½-oz. can	543	0
	1 cup (4.7 oz.)		
Canned in oil, Drained solids *(USDA)*	6½-oz. can	309	0
Albacore *(Del Monte)*	1 cup (5.6 oz.)	306	0
Chunk light *(Chicken of The Sea)*	6½-oz. can	294	0
(Del Monte)	1 cup (5.6 oz.)	374	0
(Icy Point)	6½-oz. can	280	0
(Pillar Rock)	6½-oz. can	280	0
(Snow Mist)	6½-oz. can	280	0
Solid white *(Icy Point)*	7-oz. can	286	0
(Pillar Rock)	7-oz. can	286	0
Canned in water, Solids & Liquid *(USDA)*	6½-oz. can	234	0
(Breast O'Chicken)	6½-oz. can	230	0
(Star-Kist)	7-oz. can	210	0
Canned in water, Drained, Solid, light *(Chicken of The Sea)*	6½-oz. can	224	0
White *(Chicken of The Sea)*	6½-oz. can	216	0
Canned, dietetic, Drained, Chunk ,white *(Chicken of The Sea)*	6½-oz. can	200	0
Solids & liquid *(Star-Kist)*	6½-oz. can	207	0
(Star-Kist)	3¼-oz. can	112	0
Tuna Helper, Creamy noodles 'n' tuna *(Betty Crocker)*	1/5 pkg., (6½ oz.) tuna	280	30
Tuna Helper, Creamy rice 'n' Tuna *(Betty Crocker)*	1/5 pkg. plus 1/5 can (6½ oz.) tuna	250	33

E
F

119

Food and Description	Measure or Quantity	Cal-ories	Carbo-hydrates (grams)
Tuna & Noodle dinner (Star-Kist)	15-oz. can	364	
Tuna Salad, Home recipe, Made with tuna, celery, mayonnaise, pickle, onion & egg (USDA)	4 oz.	193	4.0
Turbot, Raw, whole, Greenland (USDA)	1 lb. (weighed whole	344	0
Meat only (USDA)	4 oz.	166	0
FLAVORINGS, SEASONINGS			
Almond Extract (Ehlers)	1 tsp.	5	
(French's)	1-tsp.	12	
Anise Extract (Ehlers)	1 tsp.	12	
(French's)	1 tsp.	26	
Bacon Bits, Imitation (Durkee)	1 tsp. (2 grams)	8	.5
(French's)	1 tsp. (2 grams)	7	.4
(McCormick)	1 oz.	113	7.7
Bacos * (General Mills)	1 tbsp.	29	1.0
Banana Extract, Imitation (Ehlers)	1 tsp.	7	
(French's)	1 tsp.	20	
Barbecue Dinner Mix, Skillet (Hunt's)	2-lb. 1-oz. pkg.	1404	271.1
Beef, Ground, Seasoning mix (Durkee)	1-1/8-oz. pkg.	92	19.9
With onions (French's)	1-1/8-oz. pkg.	79	17.5
Beef Goulash Seasoning mix (Lawry's)	1.7-oz. pkg.	127	24.1

*Prepared as package directs.

Food and Description	Measure or Quantity	Calories	Carbo-hydrates (grams)
Butter, Imitation (Ehlers)	1 tsp.	7	
(French's)	1 tsp.	8	
Maple (Ehlers)	1 tsp.	9	
(French's)	1 tsp.	9	
Marinade mix, Beef (Lawry's)	1.6-oz. pkg.	69	15.1
Instant, meat (Adolph's)	.8-oz. pkg.	39	8.5
Lemon pepper (Lawry's)	2.7-oz. pkg.	159	29.7
Meat Loaf (Contadina)	3 ¾-oz. pkg.	363	70.1
(Lawry's)	3½-oz. pkg.	333	65.2
Pepper, Black (USDA)	1 cup	204	33.1
	1 tsp.	4	.7
Seasoned (French's)	1 tsp.	7	1.0
Seasoned (Lawry's)	1 pkg.	158	29.8
	1 tsp.	8	1.6
Lemon pepper (Durkee)	1 tsp.	1	.2
Pepper & lemon seasoning (French's)	1tsp.	5	1.0
Peppers, Hot, red, without seeds, dried (ground chili powder, added seasonings) (USDA)	1 tbsp.	50	8
Salad (Durkee)	1 tsp.	4	.7
With cheese (Durkee)	1 tsp.	10	.4
Salad Lift (French's)	1 tsp.	6	1.2
Salad Mate (Durkee)	1 tsp.	7	1.0
Salt, Butter flavored, imitation (Durkee)	1 tsp.	3	.2
(French's)	1 tsp.	8	
Garlic (French's)	1 tsp.	4	.7
(Lawry's)	1 tsp.	5	1.0
(Lawry's)	2.9-oz. pkg.	116	22.9
Parslied (French's)	1 tsp.	6	1.2
Hickory smoke (French's)	1 tsp.	1	Trace

E
F

Food and Description	Measure or Quantity	Cal- ories	Carbo- hydrates (grams)
Onion (French's)	1 tsp.	5	1.0
(Lawry's)	1 tsp.	4	.9
(Lawry's)	3-oz. pkg.	106	22.0
Seasoning (French's)	1 tsp.	3	.7
Seasoned (Lawry's)	1 tsp.	1	.1
(Lawry's)	3-oz. pkg.	21	2.3
Substitute (Adolph's)	1 tsp.	0	0
Seasoned (Adolph's)	1 tsp.	4	.9
Table (USDA)	1 tsp.	0	C
Seafood (French's)	1 tsp.	2	.3
Seasoned (Adolph's)	1 tsp.	2	.4
(French's)	1 tsp.	2	
Tabasco (McIlhenny)	¼ tsp.	<1	<.1
Unseasoned (Adolph's)	1 tsp.	2	.5
(French's)	1 tsp.	2	

FROZEN DINNERS

Food and Description	Measure or Quantity	Cal- ories	Carbo- hydrates (grams)
Beef Dinners (Banquet)	11 oz.	312	20.
(Morton)	10 oz.	290	20
Sliced, 3-course (Morton)	1 lb. 1 oz. dinner	563	60.
"TV" dinner (Swanson)	11½ oz.	370	34
Beef & Green Pepper Casserole (Mrs. Paul's)	12-oz. pkg.	386	31.
Beef steak & carrots (Weight Watchers)	10-oz. lun- cheon	412	8.C
Beef steak & cauliflour (Weight Watchers)	11-oz. lun- cheon	431	11.2
Chipped Beef, Creamed (Banquet)	5-oz. bag	126	9.2
Chipped Beef, Creamed, Cookin' Bag (Banquet)	5 oz.	124	10.5
Chopped beef dinner (Banquet)	11oz.	443	32.8
Chopped Sirloin beef TV Dinner (Swanson)	10 oz.	460	37

Food and Description	Measure or Quantity	Calories	Carbohydrates (grams)
Chopped beef steak, Hungry Man (Swanson)	18 oz.	730	70
Pot roast, includes whole oven-browned potatoes, peas & corn (USDA)	10 oz.	301	17.3
Beef hash, Roast (Stouffer's)	11½-oz. pkg.	460	21.7
Corned beef hash dinner (Banquet)	10 oz.	372	42.6
Beef Patties, & burgundy sauce (Morton House)	4½-oz. serving	153	8.7
& Italian sauce (Morton House)	4-1/6-oz. serving	169	12.5
& Mexican sauce (Morton House)	4-1/6-oz. serving	155	9.0
Beef Pot Pie (Morton)	8 oz.	390	34
Beef Pie (Stouffer's)	10-oz. pkg.	572	42.9
(Swanson)	8-oz. pie	434	38.6
Deep dish (Swanson)	16-oz. pie	703	56.8
(Banquet)	8-oz. pie	411	40.5
Beef Stew, Buffet Supper Products (Banquet)	32 oz.	700	90.9
Gravy and Sliced Beef (Morton House)	6¼ oz.	190	8
Cookin' Bag (Banquet)	5 oz.	116	4.8
Buffet Supper (Banquet)	32 oz.	782	34.5
Sliced Beef Country Table Dinner (Morton)	14 oz.	560	57
Blintze, Apple, Blueberry or Cherry (Aunt Leah's)	1 blintze (2.5 oz.)	80	
Cheese (Aunt Leah's)	1 blintze (2.5 oz.)	70	
Chicken, Boneless chicken dinner (Morton)	10 oz.	260	22

EF

Food and Description	Measure or Quantity	Calories	Carbo-hydrates (grams)
Chicken à la King, Cookin' Bag *(Banquet)*	5 oz.	138	10.4
Chicken croquette dinner *(Morton)*	10.25 oz.	410	45
Chicken Creole *(Weight Watchers)*	12-oz. luncheon	211	10.2
Chicken 'N Dumplings, Country Table Dinner *(Morton)*	15 oz.	580	83
Chicken & Dumplings, Buffet Supper *(Banquet)*	32 oz.	1209	128.2
Chicken 'N' Dumpling *(Morton)*	11 oz.	300	31
Chicken & Noodles Dinner *(Banquet)*	12 oz.	374	50.7
Chicken 'N Noodles Dinner *(Morton)*	10.25 oz.	260	39
Chicken Meat Pie *(Swanson)*	8 oz.	450	44
(Banquet)	8 oz.	427	39.0
Chicken Pot Pie, Baked, 4¼ in. diam., weight before baking about 8 oz.	1 pie	535	42
(Morton)	8 oz.	360	32
Creamed chicken *(Stouffer's)*	11½-oz. pkg.	613	16.2
Fried Chicken Dinner			
(Banquet)	11 oz.	530	48.4
(Morton)	11 oz.	500	46
Country Table Dinner *(Morton)*	15 oz.	740	70
"TV" Dinner *(Swanson)*	11½ oz.	570	448
Man Pleaser *(Banquet)*	17 oz.	916	89.2
Clams, Clams Casino *(Mrs. Paul's)*	two	220	19
Clams Rockefeller *(Mrs. Paul's)*	two	260	19
Clam sticks *(Mrs. Paul's)*	five	240	32
Clam thins *(Mrs. Paul's)*	two	310	32
Deviled clams *(Mrs. Paul's)*	one	180	14
Fried clams *(Mrs. Paul's)*	2½ oz.	270	25

Food and Description	Measure or Quantity	Calories	Carbohydrates (grams)
Crab, Thawed & drained, Alaska			
King *(Wakefield's)*	4 oz.	96	.6
Deviled crab *(Mrs. Paul's)*	one	160	18
Crab miniatures *(Mrs. Paul's)*	3½ oz.	220	26
Deviled *(Mrs. Paul's)*	4 oz.	230	
Newburg *(Stouffer's)*	12-oz. pkg.	562	13.6
Enchilada, Beef, 3 compartments,			
Complete dinner *(Banquet)*	12 oz.	467	61.0
(Patio)	13 oz.	320	34.0
Complete dinner *(Swanson)*	15 oz.	561	59.5
5 compartments, Complete Dinner *(Patio)*	13 oz.	610	93.0
Enchilada, Cheese, 3 compartments,			
Complete dinner *(Banquet)*	12½ oz.	482	58.2
(Patio)	12 oz.	330	40.0
5 compartments, Complete Dinner *(Patio)*	12 oz.	380	55.0
Fish cake *(Mrs. Paul's)*	two	210	23
Fish Dinner, *(Banquet)*	8¾ oz.	382	43.6
(Morton)	8¾ oz.	375	42.4
With green beans & peach *(Weight Watchers)*	18 oz.	266	21.9
With pineapple chunks *(Weight Watchers)*	9½-oz. (luncheon)	175	17.2
Filet of Ocean Fish "TV" Dinner *(Swanson)*	11½ oz.	440	38
Filet of Ocean Fish with French Fries *(Swanson)*	9¾ oz.	429	41.4
Fish 'n' Chips, Hungry-Man Dinner *(Swanson)*	15¾ oz.	760	68
"TV" Dinner *(Swanson)*	10¼ oz.	450	40
Fish sticks *(Mrs. Paul's)*	four	150	16
Breaded, cooked; stick 3¾ by 1 by ½ in.	8-oz. pkg. or 10 sticks	400	15

E
F

Food and Description	Measure or Quantity	Calories	Carbohydrates (grams)
Flounder, fillets (Mrs. Paul's)	two	220	22
Frankfurter & Bean, Complete Dinner.	11½ oz.	610	70.1
Complete Dinner (Morton)	12 oz.	554	81.3
Meat compartment.	6¼ oz.	481	30.2
Apple compartment.	2½ oz.	77	18.2
Cornbread compartment.	2 oz.	129	22.0
Complete dinner (Banquet)	10 ¾-oz. dinner	687	70.5
Franks, Beans and franks dinner (Banquet)	10 ¾ oz.	528	63.1
(Morton)	10.75 oz.	540	79
German Dinner (Swanson)	11 oz.	405	42.2
Haddock, dinner (Banquet)	8¾ oz.	419	45.4
(Morton)	9 oz.	350	24
Haddock fillets (Mrs. Paul's)	two	230	24
Lobster Newburg (Stouffer's)	11½-oz. pkg.	671	16.0
Meat Loaf Dinner (Morton)	11 oz.	370	28
(Banquet)	11 oz.	412	29.0
Country Table Dinner (Morton)	15 oz.	520	61
"TV" Dinner (Swanson)	10 ¾ oz.	530	48
Meat Loaf, Man Pleaser (Banquet)	19 oz.	916	63.6
Meat Loaf Cookin' Bag (Banquet)	5 oz.	224	13.6
Mushroom Gravy & Salisbury Steak (Morton House)	4-1/16 oz.	160	7
Ocean Perch, dinner (Banquet)	8 ¾ oz.	434	49.8
Oysters (Ship Ahoy)	10-oz. pkg.	239	5.0
Perch, Breaded (Gorton)	⅓ of 11-oz. pkg.	113	9.0
Pizza, Cheese, 5½ in. sector, 1/8 of 14 in. diam. pie (USDA)	1 sector	185	27
Cheese pizza (Celeste)	¼ of 20-oz. pizza	321	35.6

Food and Description	Measure or Quantity	Calories	Carbohydrates (grams)
Sausage pizza *(Celeste)*	¼ of 23-oz. pizza	400	38
Pork dinners, Loin of pork "TV" dinner *(Swanson)*	11¼ oz.	470	48
Ham dinner, cured, cooked *(Banquet)*	10 oz.	369	47.7
Ham dinner *(Morton)*	10 oz.	450	57
Ham "TV" dinner *(Swanson)*	10 ¼ oz.	380	47
Gravy and sliced pork *(Morton House)*	6¼ oz.	190	9
Salisbury Steak *(Swanson)*	11½ oz.	500	40
(Morton)	11 oz.	320	25
Salmon, Steak *(Ship Ahoy)*	12-oz. pkg.	405	0
Scallops, Breaded, fried, re-heated *(USDA)*	4 oz.	220	11.9
(Mrs. Paul's)	3½ oz.	210	24
Crisps *(Gorton)*	½ of 7-oz. pkg.	155	8.0
Sole *(Gorton)*	1/3 of 1 lb. pkg.	120	0
Fillet, thawed *(Ship Ahoy)*	1-lb. pkg.	309	0
Fillets *(Mrs. Paul's)*	two	220	22
In Lemon butter *(Gorton)*	1/3 of 9-oz. pkg.	147	2.0
Shrimp, Unbreaded *(Chicken of The Sea)*	4 oz.	103	
Cooked *(Sau-Sea)*	4 oz.	73	0
Cooked *(Weight Watchers)*	4 oz. (½ pkg.)	67	1.3
Fried *(Chicken of The Sea)*	4 oz.	255	
Fried *(Mrs. Paul's)*	3 oz.	170	17
Scampi *(Gorton)*	½ of 7-oz. pkg.	285	7.0
Raw, breaded *(Gorton)*	¼ of 1-lb. pkg.	158	23.0
Raw, peeled *(Ship Ahoy)*	8-oz. pkg.	207	1.5
Shrimp cake, Fried, breaded *(Mrs. Paul's)*	1 cake	158	6.0

E
F

Food and Description	Measure or Quantity	Calories	Carbohydrates (grams)
Shrimp cake, Thins (Mrs. Paul's)	10-oz. pkg.	630	61.3
Shrimp "TV" dinner (Swanson)	8 oz.	360	47
Shrimp dinner (Morton)	7.75 oz.	400	38
Spaghetti Dinners, Spaghetti & Meatballs (Banquet)	11½ oz.	450	62.9
(Morton)	11 oz.	360	59
(Swanson)	12½ oz.	410	57
Swiss Steak "TV" Dinner (Swanson)	10 oz.	350	40
Tuna Cake, Thins (Mrs. Paul's)	10-oz. pkg.	689	47.1
Tuna Meat Pie (Banquet)	8 oz.	434	42.7
Tuna Pot Pie (Morton)	8 oz.	400	39
Tuna Pie (Banquet)	8-oz. pie	479	40.2
(Morton)	8-oz. pie	385	35.8
(Star-Kist)	8-oz. pie	450	
Turbot (Weight Watchers)	18-oz. dinner	426	17.4
With apple (Weight Watchers)	9½-oz. luncheon	277	11.0
Turkey Dinner (Banquet)	11 oz.	293	27.8
(Morton)	11 oz.	470	47
Hungry Man Turkey dinner (Swanson)	19 oz.	740	80
Man-Pleaser dinner (Banquet)	19 oz.	620	73.8
Turkey Tetrazzini dinner (Morton)	11½ oz.	360	45
"TV" dinner (Swanson)	11½ oz.	360	45
Turkey Meat Pie (Banquet)	8 oz.	415	40.6
(Swanson)	8 oz.	450	40
Turkey Pot Pie (Morton)	8 oz.	400	32
Sliced Turkey Country dinner (Morton)	15 oz.	640	82
Veal Parmigiana (Banquet)	11 oz.	421	42.1
Cookin' Bag (Banquet)	5 oz.	287	19.5
Hungry Man Veal Parmigiana Dinner (Swanson)	20½ oz.	910	70
"TV" dinner (Swanson)	12½ oz.	520	47

FRUITS

Food and Description	Measure or Quantity	Calories	Carbohydrates (grams)
Apples, any variety, Fresh,			
Eaten with skin *(USDA)*	1 med.-2½ in. diam. (about 3 per lb.)	80	20.0
Pared, diced.	1 cup	59	15.4
Apples, raw (about 3 per lb.) *(USDA)*	1 apple	70	18
Evaporated, uncooked *(Del Monte)*	2 oz.	140	37
Sliced apples, packed with water and sugar *(White House)*	4 oz.	54	14
Spiced apple rings *(White House)*	1 apple ring	19	5
Applesauce, canned, sweetened *(USDA)*	1 cup	230	61
Canned, unsweetened, or artificially sweetened *(USDA)*	1 cup	100	26
(Del Monte)	1 cup	170	47
(S & W Nutradiet)	½ cup	55	14
Regular or Chunky *(White House)*	4 oz.	103	27
Dietetic *(White House)*	4 oz.	50	12
Apricots, raw, about 12 per lb. *(USDA)*	3 apricots	55	14
Canned in heavy syrup *(USDA)*	1 cup	220	57
Halves, unpeeled *(Del Monte)*	1 cup	200	52
Halves *(S & W Nutradiet)*	½ cup	35	9
Whole, peeled *(Del Monte)*	1 cup	200	53
Solids & liquid, heavy syrup *(Libby's)*	1 cup	200	54
Cooked, unsweetened, fruit and liquid *(USDA)*	1 cup	240	62
Dried, uncooked, 40 halves per cup *(USDA)*	1 cup	390	100
Dried, uncooked *(Del Monte)*	2 oz.	140	35

Food and Description	Measure or Quantity	Calories	Carbohydrates (grams)
Avocados, whole fruit, raw, California, mid & late winter; 3-1/8 in. diam. *(USDA)*	1 avocado	370	13
Florida, late summer, fall; 3-5/8 in. diam. *(USDA)*	1 avocado	390	27
California varieties, peeled pitted, mashed *(USDA)*	½ cup (4.1 oz.)	194	7.3
Florida varieties, peeled, pitted, mashed *(USDA)*	½ cup (4.1 oz.)	194	7.3
California varieties	½ avocado (3-1/8 in. diam.)	185	6.5
Florida varieties	½ avocado (3-5/8 in. diam.)	195	13.4
Bananas, Common, fresh, whole *(USDA)*	1 lb. (weighed with skin)	262	68.5
Large size *(USDA)*	7-oz. banana (9-¾ in. × 1-7/16 in.)	116	30.2
Medium size *(USDA)*	1 banana	100	26
Small size *(USDA)*	4.9-oz. banana (7-¾ in. × 1-11/32 in.)	81	21.1
Chunks *(USDA)*	1 cup (5 oz.)	122	31.7
Mashed *(USDA)*	1 cup (2 med., 7.8 oz.)	189	49.3
Sliced *(USDA)*	1 cup (1¼ med., 5.1 oz.)	124	32.4

Food and Description	Measure or Quantity	Calories	Carbohydrates (grams)
Small size (Del Monte)	1 peeled (3.5 oz.)	84	21.1
Red, peeled (USDA)	4 oz.	102	26.5
Red, whole (USDA)	1 lb. (weighed with skin)	278	72.2
Banana flakes (USDA)	1 cup	340	89
Dehydrated, powder (USDA)	1 oz.	96	25.1
Blackberries, raw (USDA)	1 cup	85	19
Canned regular, solids, light syrup (USDA)	4 oz.	82	19.6
Canned, water pack, solid & liquid (USDA)	¼ cup (4.3 oz.)	49	11.0
Canned, low calorie, solids & liquid (S & W Nutradiet)	4 oz.	41	11.2
Frozen, sweetened, not thawed (USDA)	4 oz.	109	27.7
Blueberries, raw (USDA)	1 cup	85	21
Canned, water pack (USDA)	½ cup (4.3 oz.)	47	11.9
Frozen, unsweetened, solids & liquid (USDA)	½ cup (2.9 oz.)	45	11.2
Frozen, sweetened, solids & liquid (USDA)	½ cup	120	30.2
Frozen, Quick Thaw (Bird's Eye)	½ cup (5 oz.)	114	28.7
Canteloupe, Fresh, whole (USDA)	1 lb. (weighed whole)	68	17.0
Raw, med., 5 in. diam., about 1-2/3 lbs.	½ melon	60	14
Fresh, cubed (USDA)	½ cup	24	6.1
Casaba Melon, Fresh, flesh only (USDA)	4 oz.	31	7.4

E
F

131

Food and Description	Measure or Quantity	Calories	Carbohydrates (grams)
Whole (USDA)	1 lb. (weighed whole)	61	14.7
Coconut, Fresh, whole, meat only (USDA)	4 oz.	392	10.7
Grated or shredded (USDA)	1 firmly-packed cup (4.6 oz.)	450	12.2
Grated (USDA)	1 lightly-packed cup (2.9 oz.)	277	7.5
Milk liquid expressed from mixture of grated coconut & water (USDA)	4 oz.	286	5.9
Water liquid from coconut (USDA)	1 cup	53	11.3
Dried, canned, or packaged, Sweetened, shredded (USDA)	½ lightly-packed cup	252	24.5
Unsweetened (USDA)	½ lightly-packed cup	305	10.6
Angel Flake (Baker's)	½ cup	178	14.8
Cookie (Baker's)	½ cup	280	23.2
Crunchies (Baker's)	½ cup	352	20.6
Premium shred (Baker's)	½ cup	210	18.2
Southern style (Baker's)	½ cup	170	14.8
Cherries, Fresh, sour, whole (USDA)	1 lb. (weighed without stems)	242	59.7
Pitted (USDA)	½ cup (2.7 oz.)	45	11.0
Sweet, whole, with stems (USDA)	½ cup (2.3 oz.)	41	10.2

Food and Description	Measure or Quantity	Calories	Carbo-hydrates (grams)
Pitted *(USDA)*	½ cup (2.9 oz.)	57	14.3
Canned, dark, sweet with pits *(Del Monte)*	1 cup	180	48
Canned, pitted, dark, sweet *(Del Monte)*	1 cup	190	50
Canned, dark, sweet *(S & W Nutradiet)*	½ cup	70	17
Canned, red, sour, pitted, waterpack *(USDA)*	1 cup	105	26
Canned, light, sweet, with pits, Royal Anne *(Del Monte)*	1 cup	190	51
Canned, Royal Anne, water pack *(S & W Nutradiet)*	½ cup	70	17
Candied *(USDA)*	1 oz.	96	24.6
(Liberty)	1 oz.	93	22.6
Citron, Candied *(USDA)*	1 oz.	89	22.7
(Liberty)	1 oz.	93	22.6
Cranberries, Fresh fruit *(Ocean Spray)*	2 oz. (½ cup)	25	6
Cranberry Orange Relish *(Ocean Spray)*	2 oz.	100	26
Cranberry sauce, sweetened, Canned, strained *(USDA)*	1 cup	405	104
Jellied cranberry sauce *(Ocean Spray)*	2 oz.	90	22
Whole cranberry sauce *(Ocean Spray)*	2 oz.	90	21
Currants, zante *(Del Monte)*	½ cup	190	48
Dates, pitted, cut *(USDA)*	1 cup	490	130
Dry, Domestic, with pits *(USDA)*	1 lb. (weighed with pits)	1081	287.7
Dry, domestic, without pits *(USDA)*	4 oz.	311	82.7
(Dromedary)	1 cup	470	112.3

Food and Description	Measure or Quantity	Calories	Carbohydrates (grams)
Dry, domestic, whole (Cal-Date)	1 date	62	16.4
Figs, Fresh (USDA)	1 lb.	363	92.1
Small (USDA)	1½-in. fig	30	7.7
Canned, whole (Del Monte)	1 cup	210	55
Canned, regular pack, light syrup, solids & liquid (USDA)	4 oz.	74	19.1
Canned, heavy syrup, solids & liquid (Stokely-Van Camp)	½ cup	100	26.1
Canned, unsweetened, or dietetic pack, Kadota, solids & liquid (Tillie Lewis)	½ cup	76	18.2
Canned, whole, low calorie (S & W Nutradiet)	6 figs	49	12.1
Dried, chopped, 2 in. by 1 in. (USDA)	1 cup	469	118.2
Dried, Mission (Del Monte)	1 cup	380	93.5
Fruit cocktail, Canned in heavy syrup (USDA)	1 cup	195	50
(Del Monte)	1 cup	170	45
(Libby's)	1 cup	178	46.8
(S & W Nutradiet)	½ cup	40	10
Fruits for salad (Del Monte)	1 cup	170	46
(Libby's)	1 cup	180	48
(S & W Nutradiet)	½ cup	50	11
Fruit salad, tropical (Del Monte)	1 cup	200	52
Grapefruit, raw, medium, 3-¾ in. diam. (USDA)	½ grape-fruit	45	12
Pink or red (USDA)	½ grape-fruit	50	13
Canned, syrup pack (USDA)	1 cup	180	45
Sections in juice (Del Monte)	1 cup	90	21
Sections in syrup (Del Monte)	1 cup	140	35

Food and Description	Measure or Quantity	Calories	Carbo-hydrates (grams)
Juice pack (S & W Nutradiet)	½ cup	40	9
Grapefruit Peel, Candied			
(USDA)	1 oz.	90	22.9
(Liberty)	1 oz.	93	22.6
Grapes, raw, American type,			
slip skin (USDA)	1 cup	65	15
European type, adherent skin			
(USDA)	1 cup	95	25
Honeydew, Fresh, wedge (USDA)	2 in. × 7 in.	31	7.2
Flesh only, diced (USDA)	1 cup	55	12.9
Kumquat, Fresh, whole (USDA)	1 lb. (weighed with seeds)	274	72.1
Flesh & skin (USDA)	4 oz.	74	19.4
Lemons, raw, 2-1/8 in. diam., size 165 used for juice (USDA)	1 lemon	20	6
Lemon juice, raw (USDA)	1 cup	60	20
Lemon peel, Candied (USDA)	1 oz.	90	22.9
(Liberty)	1 oz.	93	22.6
Lime juice, Fresh (USDA)	1 cup	65	22
Canned, unsweetened (USDA)	1 cup	65	22
Mixed fruit, Frozen (Bird's Eye)	5 oz.	130	34
Mandarin Orange, Canned, light syrup (Del Monte)	½ cup	77	20.6
Canned, low calorie, solids & liquid (Diet Delight)	½ cup	31	7.4
Canned, unsweetened, solids & liquid (S & W Nutradiet)	4 oz.	31	7.1
Mango, Fresh, whole (USDA)	1 med. (7.1 oz.)	88	22.5
Flesh only, diced or sliced (USDA)	½ cup	54	13.8
Oranges, raw, 2-5/8 in. diam., all commercial varieties (USDA)	1 orange	65	16

E
F

Food and Description	Measure or Quantity	Calories	Carbohydrates (grams)
Orange Peel, Candied (USDA)	1 oz.	90	22.9
(Liberty)	1 oz.	93	22.6
Papaya, Fresh, whole (USDA)	1 lb. (weighed with skin & seeds)	119	30.4
Flesh only (USDA)	4 oz.	44	11.3
Cubed (USDA)	1 cup	71	18.2
Peaches, raw, whole, medium, 2 in. diam., about 4 per lb. (USDA)	1 peach	35	10
Raw, sliced (USDA)	1 cup	65	16
Canned, yellow-fleshed, solids & liquid, syrup pack, halves or slices (USDA)	1 cup	200	52
Canned, water pack (USDA)	1 cup	75	20
Canned, cling, solids & liquid, heavy syrup (Libby's)	1 cup	170	45
Canned, cling halves (S & W Nutradiet)	½ cup	30	8
Canned, freestone halves or slices (Del Monte)	1 cup	170	45
Canned, spiced with pits (Del Monte)	7¼ oz.	150	40
Canned, yellow cling, halves or slices (Del Monte)	1 cup	170	45
Canned (Hunt-Wesson)	1 cup	192	50.4
Dried, uncooked (USDA)	1 cup	420	109
(Del Monte)	2 oz.	140	35
Dried, cooked, unsweetened, 10 to 12 halves & juice (USDA)	1 cup	220	58
Frozen, 12-oz. carton, not thawed (USDA)	1 carton	300	77
Frozen (Bird's Eye)	5 oz.	130	34
Pears, Raw, 3 in. by 2½ in. diam. (USDA)	1 pear	100	25
Canned, solids & liquid, syrup			

Food and Description	Measure or Quantity	Calories	Carbohydrates (grams)
pack, heavy, halves or slices (USDA)	1 cup	195	50
Canned, Bartlett halves or slices (Del Monte)	1 cup	160	43
Canned (Hunt-Wesson)	1 cup	181	46.3
Canned, solids & liquid, heavy syrup (Libby's)	1 cup	170	44
Halves, water pack (S & W Nutradiet)	½ cup	40	10
Dry, uncooked (Del Monte)	2 oz.	150	40
Persimmon, Japanese or Kaki, Fresh, with seeds (USDA)	1 lb. (weighed with skin, calyx & seeds)	286	73.3
(USDA)	4.4-oz. persimmon	79	20.1
Seedless (USDA)	4.4-oz. persimmon	81	20.7
Native, fresh, whole (USDA)	1 lb. (weighed with calyx & seeds)	472	124.6
Native, fresh, flesh only (USDA)	4 oz.	144	38.0
Pineapple, Raw, diced (USDA)	1 cup	75	19
Canned, heavy syrup pack, solids & liquid, crushed (USDA)	1 cup	195	50
Crushed chunks or medium slices in juice (Del Monte)	1 cup	140	35
Crushed, chunks or medium slices in syrup (Del Monte)	1 cup	190	49
Sliced, juice pack (S & W Nutradiet)	1 slice	70	17

E F

Food and Description	Measure or Quantity	Calories	Carbo-hydrates (grams)
Sliced, Slices & juice (USDA)	2 small or 1 large slice	90	24
Tidbits, juice pack (S & W Nutradiet)	½ cup	70	17
Plums, All except prunes, raw, 2 in. diam., about 2 oz. (USDA)	1 plum	25	7
Canned, syrup pack (Italian Prunes) with pits & juice (USDA)	1 cup	205	53
Purple with pits (Del Monte)	1 cup	190	52
Purple plums, water pack (S & W Nutradiet)	½ cup	55	17
Prunes, Cooked, unsweetened, 17-18 prunes & 1/3 cup liquid (USDA)	1 cup	295	78
Dried, "softenized," medium, uncooked (USDA)	4 prunes	70	18
Dried, uncooked with pits (Del Monte)	2 oz.	120	31
Dry, pitted (Del Monte)	2 oz.	140	36
Stewed, with pits (Del Monte)	1 cup	230	60
Raisins, Seedless, ½ oz. or 1½ tbsp. per pkg. (USDA)	1 pkg.	40	11
Cup pressed down (USDA)	1 cup	480	128
Golden seedless (Del Monte)	3 oz.	260	68
Muscat (Del Monte)	3 oz.	250	66
Raspberries, Red, raw (USDA)	1 cup	70	17
Frozen, 10-oz. carton, not thawed (USDA)	1 carton	275	70
Frozen (Bird's Eye)	5 oz.	140	35
Rhubarb, Cooked, sugar added (USDA)	1 cup	385	98
Strawberries, Raw, capped (USDA)	1 cup	55	13
Canned, water pack (S & W Nutradiet)	½ cup	35	7
Frozen, 10-oz. carton, not thawed (USDA)	1 carton	310	79
Frozen, sliced (Bird's Eye)	5 oz.	180	48

Food and Description	Measure or Quantity	Cal- ories	Carbo- hydrates (grams)
Frozen, whole (Bird's Eye)	4 oz.	80	23
Frozen, halves Bird's Eye)	5.3 oz.	170	48
Tangerines, Raw, medium, 2-3/8 in. diam., size 176 (USDA)	1 tangerine	40	10
Fresh, Peeled (Sunkist)	4.1 oz.	39	10.0
Watermelon, Raw, wedge 4 in. by 8 in. (USDA)	1 wedge	115	27

GELATIN

Food and Description	Measure or Quantity	Cal- ories	Carbo- hydrates (grams)
Gelatin Desserts (Royal)	½ cup	80	18.9
Low calorie (D-Zerta)	½ cup	8	0
Powder package (USDA)	1 3-oz. pkg.	315	75
Dessert powder, Prepared with fruit added *(Royal)	½ cup	82	18.4
Dessert powder, Prepared with fruit added *(USDA)	½ cup	81	19.8
Plain dry powder in envelope (USDA)	1 envelope	25	0
Prepared with water (USDA)	1 cup	140	34
Prepared with water, cherry (Jello)	½ cup	80	18
Prepared with water, straw- berry (Jello)	½ cup	80	19
Unflavored (Knox)	1 envelope	25	0

GRAIN PRODUCTS

Food and Description	Measure or Quantity	Cal- ories	Carbo- hydrates (grams)
Barley, Pearled, light, uncooked (USDA)	1 cup	700	158
Pearled (Quaker Scotch Brand)	1 cup cooked	173	37.4
Pearled, quick cooking (Quaker Scotch Brand)	¾ cup cooked	173	37.4
Cornmeal, Enriched, uncooked, degerminated (Quaker or Aunt Jemima)	¼ cup	101	22.2

*Prepared as package directs.

Food and Description	Measure or Quantity	Calories	Carbohydrates (grams)
Enriched, uncooked, bolted (Quaker or Aunt Jemima)	¼ cup	102	21.2
Enriched, degermed, cooked (USDA)	1 cup	120	26
Corn Starch (Argo Kingsford & Duryea's)	1 tbsp.	35	8
Flour, All purpose flour (Pillsbury)	1 cup	400	87
All purpose or family flour, enriched, unsifted (USDA)	1 cup	455	95
Sifted (USDA)	1 cup	420	88
Buckwheat flour, light, sifted (USDA)	1 cup	340	78
Cake or pastry flour, sifted (USDA)	1 cup	350	76
Plain flour (Ballard)	1 cup	400	87
Self-rising, enriched flour (Aunt Jemima)	¼ cup	96	20.8
(USDA)	1 cup	440	93
Self-rising flour (Ballard)	1 cup	380	84
(Pillsbury)	1 cup	380	84
Self-rising cake flour (Presto)	¼ cup	100	21
Whole-wheat flour (Pillsbury)	1 cup	400	80
Whole-wheat flour from hard wheats, stirred (USDA)	1 cup	400	85
Macaroni, Cooked, Enriched, Firm stage (undergoes additional cooking in a food mixture) (USDA)	1 cup	190	39
Cooked, Unenriched, Firm (undergoes additional cooking in a food mixture (USDA)	1 cup	190	39
Cooked until tender, enriched (USDA)	1 cup	155	32

Food and Description	Measure or Quantity	Calories	Carbohydrates (grams)
Cooked until tender, unenriched (USDA)	1 cup	155	32
Enriched (San Giorgio)	2 oz. dry	210	42
Macaroni Dinners, Macaroni 'n Beef in tomato sauce, canned (Franco-American)	7½ oz.	220	27
Macaroni & beef, frozen			
(Banquet)	12 oz.	394	55.1
(Morton)	11 oz.	310	47
(Swanson)	12 oz.	400	56
Macaroni & cheddar casserole mix (Betty Crocker)	¼ pkg.	220	35
Macaroni (enriched) & cheese, baked (USDA)	1 cup	430	40
Macaroni & cheese (Pennsylvania Dutch Brand)	½ cup	150	24
Macaroni & cheese, canned			
(USDA)	1 cup	230	26
(Franco-American)	7¼ oz.	200	26
Macaroni & cheese, frozen			
(Banquet)	12 oz.	340	45.6
(Morton)	11 oz.	350	52
(Swanson)	12½ oz.	390	55
Macaroni & cheese meat pie, frozen (Swanson)	1 pie	230	26
Noodles, Egg, cooked, enriched (USDA)	1 cup	200	37
Egg, fine, medium, broad, (Pennsylvania Dutch Brand)	2 oz.	210	40
Egg noodles plus beef sauce (Pennsylvania Dutch Brand)	½ cup	140	24
Egg noodles plus butter sauce (Pennsylvania Dutch Brand)	½ cup	150	23
Egg noodles plus cheese sauce (Pennsylvania Dutch Brand)	½ cup	150	24
Noodle products, enriched (San Giorgio)	2 oz.	220	40

G
I

Food and Description	Measure or Quantity	Calories	Carbohydrates (grams)
Noodles Almondine (*Betty Crocker*)	¼ pkg.	180	25
Noodles Romanoff (*Betty Crocker*)	¼ pkg.	160	22
Noodles Stroganoff (*Betty Crocker*)	¼ pkg.	170	25
Rice, White, enriched, raw (*USDA*)	1 cup	670	149
White, cooked (*USDA*)	1 cup	225	50
White, enriched, parboiled (*Uncle Ben's*)	2/3 cup	121	27.6
Enriched, pre-cooked with butter (*Uncle Ben's*)	2/3 cup	126	24.2
Enriched, pre-cooked without butter or salt (*Uncle Ben's*)	2/3 cup	105	24.1
Brown, long grained, cooked without butter or salt (*Uncle Ben's*)	2/3 cup	133	28.5
Chicken flavored, dry mix, cooked without butter (*Uncle Ben's*)	½ cup	100	20.5
Fried rice mix (*Minute*)	½ cup prepared with oil	160	25
Long grain & wild rice mix (*Minute*)	½ cup prepared with butter	150	25
Spanish rice mix (*Minute*)	½ cup prepared with butter & tomatoes	150	25
Frozen, brown rice in beef stock (*Green Giant*)	1 cup	280	48
Frozen, fiesta, with corn & tomato flavoring (*Green Giant*)	1 cup	240	45

Food and Description	Measure or Quantity	Calories	Carbohydrates (grams)
Frozen, pilaf with mushrooms & onions *(Green Giant)*	1 cup	230	45
Frozen, white & wild rice *(Green Giant)*	1 cup	220	43
Spaghetti, Cooked, tender stage enriched *(USDA)*	1 cup	155	32
Spaghetti Dinners, Spaghetti with meat balls & tomato sauce, Home recipe *(USDA)*	1 cup	330	39
Spaghetti with meat balls & tomato sauce, canned *(USDA)*	1 cup	260	28
Spaghetti with meatballs in tomato sauce, canned *(Franco-American)*	7¼ oz.	230	22
Spaghetti 'n beef in tomato sauce, canned *(Franco-American)*	7½ oz.	250	28
"Spaghetti O's" with little meatballs in tomato sauce, canned *(Franco-American)*	7½ oz.	230	24
"Spaghetti O's" with sliced franks in tomato sauce, canned *(Franco-American)*	7½ oz.	240	28
Spaghetti in tomato sauce with cheese, home recipe *(USDA)*	1 cup	260	37
Spaghetti in tomato sauce with Cheese, canned *(USDA)*	1 cup	190	38
(Franco-American)	7½ oz.	180	34

G
I

GRAVY

Food and Description	Measure or Quantity	Calories	Carbohydrates (grams)
Beef, Canned *(Franco-American)*	2 oz.	35	3
Chicken, Canned *(Franco-American)*	2 oz.	55	3
Mushroom, Canned *(Franco-American)*	¼ cup	27	2.8

Food and Description	Measure or Quantity	Calories	Carbo- hydrates (grams)
Gravy Mix, Au jus (French's)	¾-oz. pkg.	44	8.7
Beef (Swiss Products)	7/8-oz. pkg.	75	15.8
Brown (Lawry's)	1¼-oz. pkg.	136	16.3
(Pillsbury)	¼ cup	15	3
(McCormick)	7/8-oz. pkg.	100	10.0
Cheese (McCormick)	1¼-oz. pkg.	170	4.8
Chicken (French's)	1¼-oz. pkg.	130	14.7
(Pillsbury)	¼ cup	30	4
Mushroom (French's)	¾-oz. pkg.	62	7.0
(Lawry's)	1.3-oz. pkg.	145	15.6
*(Wyler's)	2-oz. serving	15	1.8
Onion *(Durkee)	1 cup (1-oz. pkg.)	96	16.5
(French's)	1-oz. pkg.	72	12.3
Pork (French's)	¾-oz. pkg.	74	10.2
Turkey (French's)	7/8-oz. pkg.	90	11.5
ICE CREAM			
Any flavor, 2.5% fat (Borden)	¼ pt.	93	17.6
3.25% fat (Borden)	¼ pt.	97	18.1
Lite Line (Borden)	¼ pt.	99	16.0
Any flavor, Sweetened, 10% fat, Frozen custard or French ice cream (USDA)	1 cup	257	27.7
12% fat (USDA)	2½-oz. slice (1/8-qt. brick)	147	14.6
12% fat (USDA)	3½-fl. oz. container	128	12.8

*Prepared as package directs.

144

Food and Description	Measure or Quantity	Calories	Carbohydrates (grams)
12% fat (USDA)	1 cup (5 oz.)	294	29.3
16% fat rich (USDA)	1 cup (5.2 oz.)	329	26.6
Deluxe (Carnation)	1 cup (5 oz.)	268	32.2
Regular, Approx. 10% fat (USDA)	1 cup	255	28
	3-fl. oz. cup	95	10
Banana, Light n' Lively, (Sealtest)	¼ pt.	103	19.7
Banana Strawberry Twirl, Light n' Lively (Sealtest)	¼ pt.	111	22.1
Buttered almond, Light n' Lively (Sealtest)	¼ pt.	117	17.9
Caramel nut, Light n'Lively (Sealtest)	¼ pt.	120	18.7
Cherry Pineapple, Light n' Lively (Sealtest)	¼ pt.	98	18.8
Chocolate, 9.5% fat (Borden)	¼ pt.	126	16.9
10% fat (Meadow Gold)	¼ pt.	128	16.5
Eclair (Good Humor)	1 bar	290	33
French (Prestige)	¼ pt.	182	18.0
(Sealtest)	¼ pt.	136	17.3
Light n'Lively (Sealtest)	¼ pt.	105	19.2
Chocolate-coated, Bar (Popsicle Industries)	3-fl.-oz. bar	133	
(Popsicle Industries)	3-fl.-oz. bar	180	
(Sealtest)	2½-fl. oz. bar	149	12.1
(Sealtest)	2½-fl.-oz. bar	132	13.6
Chocolate flavor coated vanilla ice cream (Good Humor)	1 bar	310	22
Coffee, Light n'Lively (Sealtest)	¼ pt.	102	18.4

G
I

Food and Description	Measure or Quantity	Cal- ories	Carbo- hydrates (grams)
Cone only (USDA)	1 piece	19	3.9
(Comet)	1 piece	19	3.9
Assorted colors (Comet)	1 piece	19	3.9
Rolled sugar (Comet)	1 piece	49	10.2
Cup only (Comet)	1 piece	20	4.1
Assorted colors (Comet)	1 piece	20	4.1
Pilot (Comet)	1 piece	19	3.9
Hardened (USDA)	1 cup	200	29
Home recipe (USDA)	8 oz. (by wt.)	177	73.9
Lemon, Light n'Lively (Sealtest)	¼ pt.	103	18.4
Lemon chiffon, Light n'Lively (Sealtest)	¼ pt.	119	24.3
Orange pineapple, Light n' Lively (Sealtest)	¼ pt.	102	18.6
Peach, Light n'Lively (Sealtest)	¼ pt.	103	19.8
Popsicle, 3-fl.-oz. size (USDA)	1 popsicle	70	18
Raspberry, Light n'Lively (Sealtest)	¼ pt.	99	17.8
Sandwich (Sealtest)	3-fl. oz.	173	26.1
Soft-serve (USDA)	1 cup	265	39
Strawberry, Light n'Lively (Sealtest)	¼ pt.	100	18.7
Strawberry royale, Light n' Lovely (Sealtest)	¼ pt.	112	21.6
Strawberry shortcake bar (Good Humor)	1 bar	250	29
Toffee, Light n'Lively (Sealtest)	¼ pt.	110	19.1
Toffee crunch, Light n'Lively (Sealtest)	¼ pt.	119	20.2
Toasted almond (Good Humor)	1 bar	290	35
Twin Pops (Sealtest)	3-fl. oz.	70	17.9
Vanilla, 4% fat (Meadow Gold)	¼ pt.	95	16.5
Vanilla fudge royale, Light n' Lively (Sealtest)	¼ pt.	113	21.0

Food and Description	Measure or Quantity	Cal- ories	Carbo- hydrates (grams)
Vanilla, Light n'Lively (Sealtest)	¼ pt.	102	18.3
Whammy Stix. Assorted ice flavors (Good Humor)	1 bar	50	13
Chocolate (Good Humor)	1 bar	160	12
JELLIES AND PRESERVES			
Apple butter (White House)	1 tbsp.	28	7.6
(Musselman's)	1 tbsp.	33	0
(USDA)	½ cup	262	66.0
	5 oz. or 1 tbsp.	33	8.4
Apple jelly (S & W Nutradiet)	1 tsp.	3	1
Dietetic or low calorie (Diet Delight)	1 tbsp. (.6 oz.)	22	5.4
(Kraft)	1 oz.	34	8.5
Sweetened (White House)	1 tbsp. (.7 oz.)	46	13.0
Blackberry preserve or jam, Sweetened (Bama)	1 tbsp. (.7 oz.)	54	13.5
Low calorie (Diet Delight)	1 tbsp. (.6 oz.)	22	5.5
(S & W Nutradiet)	1 tbsp. (.5 oz.)	10	2.6
Cherry preserve, Sweetened (Bama)	1 tbsp.	54	13.5
Dietetic or low calorie (S & W Nutradiet)	1 tbsp. (.5 oz.)	11	2.6
Grape, Low calorie (Kraft)	1 oz.	34	8.4
(Smucker)	1 tbsp.	5	1.2
Concord (S & W Nutradiet)	1 tbsp.	10	2.5
Jelly, Sweetened (USDA)	1 tbsp.	50	13
(USDA)	1 oz.	77	20.0
All flavors (Crosse & Blackwell)	1 tbsp.	51	12.8

J M

Food and Description	Measure or Quantity	Calories	Carbohydrates (grams)
(Kraft)	1 oz.	74	18.4
(Polaner)	1 tbsp.	54	13.5
(Smucker)	1 tbsp.	49	12.4
Marmalade, Sweetened (USDA)	1 tbsp.	51	14.0
(Kraft)	1 oz.	78	19.3
Bitter or sweet (Crosse & Blackwell)	1 tbsp.	60	14.9
Low calorie (Kraft)	1 oz.	35	8.6
(S & W Nutradiet)	1 tbsp.	11	2.6
(Slenderella)	1 tbsp.	22	5.6
Peach preserve, Sweetened (Bama)	1 tbsp.	51	12.7
Low calorie or dietetic (Kraft)	1 oz.	35	8.6
(Tillie Lewis)	1 tbsp.	10	2.4
Pear preserves (Bama)	1 tbsp.	51	12.7
Preserves, Sweetened (USDA)	1 tbsp.	54	14.0
(USDA)	1 oz.	77	19.8
All flavors (Crosse & Blackwell)	1 tbsp.	59	14.8
(Kraft)	1 oz.	78	19.3
(Polaner)	1 tbsp.	54	13.5
(Smucker)	1 tbsp.	52	12.9
Plums, Damson or red, sweetened (Bama)	1 tbsp.	51	12.7
Raspberry jam, sweetened, black or red (Bama)	1 tbsp.	54	13.5
(S & W Nutradiet)	1 tsp.	4	1
Low calorie or dietetic (Diet Delight)	1 tbsp.	24	5.8
Strawberry jam, Sweetened (Bama)	1 tbsp.	54	13.5
Dietetic or low calorie (Kraft)	1 oz.	36	8.9
(S & W Nutradiet)	1 tsp.	4	1

Food and Description	Measure or Quantity	Calories	Carbo-hydrates (grams)
MEAT			
Bacon, cured, raw			
Black Label *(Hormel)*	1 piece (8 oz.)	125	.2
Range Branch *(Hormel)*	1 piece (1.6 oz.)	275	.5
(Wilson)	1 oz.	169	.3
Sliced *(USDA)*	1 lb.	3016	4.5
Slab *(USDA)*	1 lb. (weighed with rind)	2836	4.3
Sliced *(USDA)*	1 oz.	189	.3
Bacon, Broiled or fried crisp, 20 slices per lb. raw *(USDA)*	2 slices	90	1
Drained, thin slice *(USDA)*	1 slice (5 grams)	31	.2
Drained, medium slice *(USDA)*	1 slice (8 grams)	46	.2
Drained, thick slice *(USDA)*	1 slice (4 oz.)	73	.4
Drained, 11-14 slices per lb. raw *(Oscar Mayer)*	1 slice (.4 oz.)	67	.1
Drained, 18-26 slices per lb. raw *(Oscar Mayer)*	1 slice (6 grams)	36	.1
Drained, 25-30 slices per lb. raw *(Oscar Mayer)*	1 slice (4 grams)	24	.1
Bacon, cured, canned *(USDA)*	3 oz.	582	.9
Bacon, Cooked *(Oscar Mayer)*	3 slices	120	0
Bacon Bits *(Wilson)*	1 oz.	139	1.0
Bacon, Canadian, unheated *(USDA)*	1 oz.	61	Trace
(Wilson)	1 oz.	42	.1
Canadian style *(Oscar Mayer)*	2 slices	90	0
Canadian, Broiled or fried, drained *(USDA)*	1 oz.	79	Trace

J
M

Food and Description	Measure or Quantity	Calories	Carbohydrates (grams)
Beef, Cooked, Cuts braised, Simmered or pot-roasted *(USDA)*			
Lean and fat.	3 oz.	245	0
Lean only.	2.5 oz.	140	0
Beef, Brisket, raw *(USDA)*	1 lb. (weighed with bone)	1284	0
(USDA)	1 lb. (weighed without bone)	2041	0
Braised or pot-roasted, lean & fat *(USDA)*	4 oz.	467	0
Beef, Chuck, raw *(USDA)*	1 lb. (weighed with bone)	984	0
(USDA)	1 lb. (weighed without bone)	1166	0
Braised or pot-roasted, lean & fat *(USDA)*	4 oz.	371	0
Beef, Corned, uncooked, boneless, Medium fat *(USDA)*	1 lb.	1329	0
Cooked, boneless, Medium fat *(USDA)*	4 oz.	422	0
Canned, lean *(USDA)*	3 oz.	185	0
Canned, Medium fat *(USDA)*	4 oz.	245	0
Canned, fat *(USDA)*	4 oz.	298	0
Canned *(Armour Star)*	12-oz. can	967	0
Canned, Dinty Moore *(Hormel)*	4 oz.	253	0
Canned, Brisket, Tender Made *(Wilson)*	4 oz.	180	1.0
Corned beef hash, canned, with potato *(Armour Star)*	15½-oz. can	831	36.0
(Hormel)	7½ oz.	400	21.0
(Libby's)	4 oz.	192	14.3

Food and Description	Measure or Quantity	Calories	Carbohydrates (grams)
(USDA)	3 oz.	155	9
Home Style (Libby's)	4 oz.	226	13.2
(Silver Skillet)	4 oz.	217	10.9
(Wilson)	15½-oz. can	792	31.6
Beef, Chipped, uncooked (USDA)	½ cup (2.9 oz.)	166	0
(Armour Star)	1 oz.	48	0
"Slender Sliced" (Eckrich)	1 oz.	40	
Cooked, creamed, home recipe (USDA)	1 cup (8.6 oz.)	377	17.4
Cooked, thin slice (Oscar Mayer)	1 slice (5 grams)	7	.1
Canned, creamed (Swanson)	1 cup	192	11.6
Beef, Dried or chipped (USDA)	5 oz.	115	0
Beef, flank, raw, 100% lean (USDA)	1 lb.	653	0
Braised, 100% lean (USDA)	4 oz.	222	0
Beef, Ground, regular, raw (USDA)	1 lb.	1216	0
Lean, raw (USDA)	1 lb.	812	0
Broiled (USDA)	4 oz.	324	0
Broiled, Lean (USDA)	4 oz.	248	0
Broiled, Lean (USDA)	3 oz.	185	0
Regular (USDA)	3 oz.	245	0
Beef, heart, lean, braised (USDA)	3 oz.	160	1
Beef, Heel of round, raw (USDA)	1 lb.	966	0
Roasted, lean & fat (USDA)	4 oz.	296	0
Beef, Rib Roast, raw (USDA)	1 lb. (weighed with bone)	1673	0
(USDA)	1 lb. (weighed without bone)	1819	0
Roasted, lean & fat (USDA)	4 oz.	499	0

151

Food and Description	Measure or Quantity	Calories	Carbo-hydrates (grams)
Roasted, lean only *(USDA)*	4 oz.	273	0
Beef, Round, raw *(USDA)*	1 lb. (weighed without bone)	894	0
Broiled, lean only *(USDA)*	4 oz.	214	0
Beef, Rump, raw *(USDA)*	1 lb. (weighed without bone)	1374	0
Roasted, lean & fat *(USDA)*	4 oz.	393	0
Beef, Steak, Club, lean & fat Broiled *(USDA)*	4 oz.	515	0
Beef, Steak, Porterhouse, lean & fat, broiled *(USDA)*	4 oz.	527	0
Beef, Steak, Rib eye, broiled, One 10-oz. steak (weighed without bone before cooking, will give you lean & fat) *(USDA)*	7.3 oz.	911	0
Beef, Roast, oven-cooked, no liquid added, relatively fat such as Rib *(USDA)*			
Lean and fat.	3 oz.	165	0
Lean only.	2.7 oz.	125	0
Relatively lean, such as Heel of round *(USDA)*			
Lean and fat.	3 oz.	165	0
Lean only.	2.7 oz.	125	0
Beef, Salisbury steak & gravy, Cookin' Bag *(Banquet)*	5 oz.	246	7.8
Beef, Steak, Sirloin, Broiled, Lean and fat *(USDA)*	4 oz.	463	0
Lean only *(USDA)*	4 oz.	245	0
Beef, Steak, Broiled, Relatively fat, such as sirloin *(USDA)*			
Lean and fat.	3 oz.	330	0

Food and Description	Measure or Quantity	Calories	Carbohydrates (grams)
Lean only.	2.0 oz.	115	0
Relatively lean, such as round (USDA)			
Lean and fat.	3 oz.	220	0
Lean only.	2.4 oz.	130	0
Beef, Steak, T-bone, broiled			
Lean and fat (USDA)	4 oz.	536	0
Beefaroni, Canned (Chef (Boy-Ar-Dee)	1/5 of 40- -oz. can	206	27.9
Beef Goulash, Canned (Heinz)	8½-oz. can	253	20.1
Beef Hash, Roast, canned			
"Mary Kitchen" (Hormel)	7½-oz.	390	9.0
Beef Jerky, "Cow-Boy Jo's"			
(Beatrice Foods)	¼ oz.	24	.4
(General Mills)	¼ oz. (1 piece)	25	.3
Beef Pot Pie, Baked 4¼ in. diam., weight before baking about 8 oz. (USDA)	1 pie	560	43
Beef Stew, Beef and vegetable (USDA)	1 cup	210	15
Canned (Swanson)	7½ oz.	190	18
(Morton House)	8 oz.	240	17
Home recipe, made with lean beef chuck (USDA)	1 cup (8.6 oz.)	218	15.2
Canned (Armour Star)	24-oz. can	590	38.8
Canned (Dinty Moore)	8½-oz. can	193	11.6
Canned (Heinz)	8½-oz. can	253	24.2
Canned (Libby's)	8 oz.	154	15.2
Canned (Van Camp)	½ cup (4.6 oz.)	102	9.2
Beef Stroganoff, mix (Chef- -Boy-Ar-Dee)	6-2/3-oz. pkg.	232	30.6
"Skillet" (Hunt's)	1-lb. 2-oz. pkg.	794	94.0

J
M

153

Food and Description	Measure or Quantity	Calories	Carbohydrates (grams)
"Noodle-Roni"	4 oz.	126	18.6
Breakfast strips (*Morningstar*)	4 strips	100	3
Breakfast links (*Morningstar*)	3 links	180	7
Breakfast patties (*Morningstar*)	2 patties	200	8
Breakfast slices (*Morningstar*)	2 slices	130	6
Chili con carne, canned with beans (*USDA*)	1 cup	335	30
(*Swanson*)	7-¾ oz.	300	28
Without beans (*USDA*)	1 cup	510	15
Low sodium (*Swanson*)	7-¾ oz.	340	33
Chili con carne, with beans (*Morton House*)	7½ oz.	340	27
Without beans (*Morton House*)	7½ oz.	340	14
Meatball Stew (*Morton House*)	8 oz.	290	18
Meat Extenders for ground beef, Chile Tomato Hamburger Helper (*Betty Crocker*)	1/5 pkg. plus 1/5 lb. hamburger	340	29
Chile Make A Better Burger (*Lipton*)	1 pattie	170	5
Hamburger Stew Hamburger Helper (*Betty Crocker*)	1/5 pkg. plus 1/5 lb. hamburger	290	23
Hash Dinner Hamburger Helper (*Betty Crocker*)	1/5 pkg. plus 1/5 lb. hamburger	310	25
Hickory flavor Make A Better Burger (*Lipton*)	1 pattie	160	4
Pizza flavor Make A Better Burger (*Lipton*)	1 pattie	170	5
Rice Oriental Hamburger Helper (*Betty Crocker*)	1/5 pkg. plus 1/5 lb. hamburger	320	30

Food and Description	Measure or Quantity	Calories	Carbohydrates (grams)
Western Make A Better Burger (Lipton)	1 pattie	150	4
Regular Manwich (Hunt-Wesson)	15.5 oz.	243	57.9
Sloppy Joes (Morton House)	5 oz.	240	19
Frankfurter, raw, all meat (Armour Star)	1.6 oz. frank	155	0
(Hormel)	1-oz. frank (12 per 12-oz. pkg.)	90	.5
All beef (Hormel)	1.6-oz. frank (10 per 1-lb. package)	140	.6
(Hormel)	1-oz. frank (12 per 12-oz. package)	85	.4
Beef franks (Oscar Mayer)	1 link (10 per lb.)	140	1
(Eckrich)	1 frank	150	3
Jumbo franks (Eckrich)	1 frank	190	3
All meat weiners, 10 per lb. (Oscar Mayer)	1.6-oz. frank	142	1.3
Heated, 8 per lb. purchased pkg. (USDA)	1 frank	170	1
Franks, 12 oz. (Eckrich)	1 frank	120	2
16 oz. (Eckrich)	1 frank	150	3
Lamb, cooked, Lamb chop thick with bone, broiled (USDA)	4.8 oz.	400	0
Lamb chop, lean & fat (USDA)	4.0 oz.	400	0
Lamb chop, lean only (USDA)	2.6 oz.	140	0
Lamb chop, choice grade, 5-oz. chop, broiled, loin, (weighed with bone before cooking)			

J
M

155

Food and Description	Measure or Quantity	Cal- ories	Carbo- hydrates (grams)
will give you lean & fat (USDA)	2.8 oz.	280	0
Lean only (USDA)	2.3 oz.	122	0
Lamb chop, choice grade, 5-oz. rib chop, broiled, (weighed with bone before cooking)			
will give you lean & fat (USDA)	2.9 oz.	334	0
Lean only (USDA)	2 oz.	118	0
Lamb, roasted, leg, lean & fat (USDA)	3 oz.	235	0
Lean only (USDA)	2.5 oz.	130	0
Lamb, shoudler, roasted, lean & fat (USDA)	3 oz.	285	0
Lean only (USDA)	2.3 oz.	130	0
Liver, beef, fried, (USDA)	2 oz.	130	3
Calf, Fried (USDA)	4 oz.	296	4.5
Chicken, Simmered (USDA)	4 oz.	187	3.5
Goose, Raw (USDA)	1 lb.	826	24.5
Lamb, Broiled (USDA)	4 oz.	296	3.2
Turkey, Simmered, chopped (USDA)	1 cup	244	4.3
Pork, Fresh, Cooked, Pork chop, Lean only (USDA)	1.7 oz.	130	0
Pork roast, oven cooked, no liquid added, Lean & fat (USDA)	3 oz.	310	0
Lean only (USDA)	2.4 oz.	175	0
Pork cuts simmered, Lean & fat (USDA)	3 oz.	310	0
Lean only (USDA)	2.4 oz.	175	0
Pork chop, thick, with bone (USDA)	1 chop (3-5/8 oz.)	260	0
Pork chop, lean & fat (USDA)	2.3 oz.	260	0
Pork links, cooked, 16 links per lb., raw (USDA)	2 links	125	Trace

Food and Description	Measure or Quantity	Calories	Carbo-hydrates (grams)
Pork, Cured, Cooked, canned			
(USDA)	1 oz.	55	.3
(Armour Star)	1 oz.	53	0
(Hormel)	1 oz. of 1-lb. 8-oz. can	48	.2
(Hormel)	1 oz. of 6-lb. can	44	.2
Jubilee canned ham (Oscar Mayer)	4 oz.	140	0
Pork, Cured, Cooked, Ham, light cure, lean & fat, roasted			
(USDA)	3 oz.	245	0
Boneless Jubilee ham slice (Oscar Mayer)	4 oz.	160	0
Jubilee ham steaks (Oscar Mayer)	1 slice	70	0
Salt Pork, Raw, with skin (USDA)	1 lb. (weighed with skin)	3140	0
Without skin (USDA)	1 oz.	222	0
Sausage, Beef Cotto Salami (Oscar Mayer)	2 slices	100	1
Beef Summer (Oscar Mayer)	2 slices	140	1
Hard salami (Oscar Mayer)	3 slices	110	1
New England Brand (Oscar Mayer)	2 slices	60	1
Salami for beer (Oscar Mayer)	2 slices	100	1
Salami, cooked (USDA)	1 oz.	90	Trace
Salami, dry type (USDA)	1 oz.	130	Trace
Smokie Links (Oscar Mayer)	1 link	130	1
Summer (Oscar Mayer)	2 slices	150	1
Vienna, canned, 7 sausages per 5-oz. can (USDA)	1 sausage	40	Trace
Sweetbreads, Beef, raw (USDA)	1 lb.	939	0
Beef, braised (USDA)	4 oz.	363	0
Calf, raw (USDA)	1 lb.	426	0

J
M

157

Food and Description	Measure or Quantity	Calories	Carbohydrates (grams)
Calf, braised (USDA)	4 oz.	191	0
Hog, raw (USDA)	4 oz.	274	0
Lamb, raw (USDA)	1 lb.	426	0
Lamb, braised (USDA)	4 oz.	198	0
Tongue, Beef, medium fat, raw untrimmed (USDA)	1 lb.	714	1.4
Beef, medium fat, braised (USDA)	4 oz.	277	.5
Calf, raw, untrimmed (USDA)	1 lb.	454	3.1
Calf, braised (USDA)	4 oz.	181	1.1
Hog, raw, untrimmed (USDA)	1 lb.	741	1.7
Hog, braised (USDA)	4 oz.	287	.6
Lamb, raw, untrimmed (USDA)	1 lb.	659	1.7
Lamb, braised (USDA)	4 oz.	288	.6
Sheep, raw, untrimmed (USDA)	1 lb.	877	7.9
Sheep, braised (USDA)	4 oz.	366	2.7
Canned, pickled (USDA)	1 oz.	76	<.1
Canned, potted or deviled (USDA)	1 oz.	82	.2
Canned (Hormel)	1 oz. (12-oz. can)	67	<.1
Tripe, Beef, commercial (USDA)	4 oz.	113	0
Beef, Pickled (USDA)	4 oz.	70	0
Veal, Medium fat, cooked, bone removed, Veal cutlet (USDA)	3 oz.	185	
Veal roast (USDA)	3 oz.	230	0

MEATS — LUNCHEON

Food and Description	Measure or Quantity	Calories	Carbohydrates (grams)
Bar-B-Q-Loaf (Oscar Mayer)	2 slices	100	4
Bologna (Oscar Mayer)	2 slices	140	1
All meat (Armour Star)	1 oz.	99	0
(Eckrich)	1 oz.	92	
(Hormel)	1 oz.	85	.5
(Oscar Mayer) 8-10 slices per ¾ lb.	1 slice (1.3 oz.)	120	1.1

Food and Description	Measure or Quantity	Calories	Carbohydrates (grams)
8 slices per ½ lb.	1 slice (1 oz.)	89	.8
10 slices per ½ lb.	1 slice (.8 oz.)	73	.7
Garlic.	.8-oz. slice	73	.7
Beef (Oscar Mayer)	2 slices	140	1
Pure Beef (Eckrich)	1 oz.	64	
(Oscar Mayer)	1 slice (1.3 oz.)	120	1.1
Lebanon (Oscar Mayer)	.8-oz. slice	46	.9
Slice, 3 in. diam. by 1/8 in. (USDA)	2 slices	80	Trace
Braunschweiger, slice 2 in. diam. by ¼ in. (USDA)	2 slices	65	Trace
Liver Sausage (Oscar Mayer)	2 oz.	200	1
Ham, boiled, sliced (USDA)	2 oz.	135	0
Chopped (Oscar Mayer)	2 slices	130	2
Deviled, canned (USDA)	1 tbsp.	45	0
Deviled (Wm. Underwood Co.)	1 oz.	97	Trace
Ham & cheese loaf (Oscar Mayer)	2 slices	140	1
Smoked, sliced cooked ham (Oscar Mayer)	2 slices	60	0
Honey loaf (Oscar Mayer)	2 slices	80	2
Liverwurst spread (Wm. Underwood Co.)	1 oz.	92	1.1
Liver Cheese (Oscar Mayer)	2 slices	210	2
Luncheon Meat (Oscar Mayer)	2 slices	200	2
Canned, spice or unspiced (USDA)	2 oz.	165	1
Old Fashioned Loaf (Oscar Mayer)	2 slices	130	5
Olive Loaf (Oscar Mayer)	2 slices	130	6
Pickle & Pimento Loaf (Oscar Mayer)	2 slices	130	7
Sandwich Spread (Oscar Mayer)	2 oz.	130	7

J
M

Food and Description	Measure or Quantity	Calories	Carbohydrates (grams)
MILK & MILK PRODUCTS			
Buttermilk, Dried, packaged			
(USDA)	1 cup	465	60
Fluid, cultured, made from			
skim milk (USDA)	1 cup	90	12
Cultured, Fresh (USDA)	1 cup	88	12.5
0.5% fat (Meadow Gold)	1 cup	105	12.0
1.0% fat (Borden)	1 cup	88	12.4
0.1% fat (Borden)	1 cup	107	12.4
3.5% fat (Borden)	1 cup	159	12.0
Golden Nugget (Sealtest)	1 cup	92	10.0
Light N'Lively (Sealtest)	1 cup	95	10.5
Lowfat (Sealtest)	1 cup	114	9.3
Skim milk (Sealtest)	1 cup	71	9.3
Canned, Concentrated, Undiluted,			
Condensed, sweetened (USDA)	1 cup	980	166
Evaporated, unsweetened			
(USDA)	1 cup	345	24
Chocolate, Fresh, with whole			
milk (USDA)	1 cup	212	27.5
3.3% milkfat (Meadow Gold)	1 cup	200	27.0
3.4 fat (Sealtest)	1 cup	207	25.9
With skim milk, 2% fat			
(Meadow Gold)	1 cup	185	27.0
0.5% fat (Sealtest)	8 fl. oz. (8.6 oz.)	146	26.2
1% fat (Sealtest)	8 fl. oz. (8.6 oz.)	158	26.2
2% fat (Sealtest)	8 fl. oz. (8.6 oz.)	178	26.1
Chocolate flavored beverage			
powder with nonfat dried			
milk (USDA)	1 oz.	100	20
Chocolate flavored drink,			
Made with skim milk and 2%			
added butterfat (USDA)	1 cup	190	27
Condensed, Sweetened, canned			
(Borden)	14-oz. can	1300	218.3

Food and Description	Measure or Quantity	Cal- ories	Carbo- hydrates (grams)
Dime Brand	1 fl. oz.	125	21.1
(Eagle Brand)	1 fl. oz.	125	21.1
(Magnolia Brand)	1 fl. oz.	125	21.1
Cream, Half & Half, cream and milk (USDA)	1 tbsp.	20	1
(USDA)	1 cup	325	11
10.5% fat (Sealtest)	1 cup	296	10.2
12% fat (Sealtest)	1 cup	322	10.0
12.8% fat (Meadow Gold)	1 cup	480	9.6
	1 tbsp.	30	.6
Imitation Cream Products, Creamer, liquid (frozen) (USDA)	1 cup	345	25
	1 tbsp.	20	2
Creamer, powdered (USDA)	1 cup	505	52
	1 tbsp.	10	1
Substitute, Coffee-mate (Carnation)	1 tsp.	11	1.0
	1 packet	17	1.7
Substitute, Coffee Rich	1 tsp.	8	.7
Substitute, Coffee Twin (Sealtest)	½ fl. oz.	15	.9
Substitute, Cremora (Borden)	1 tsp.	11	1.1
Substitute, Half & Half (Meadow Gold)	1 tsp.	9	.4
Substitute, Pream.	1 tsp.	11	1.1
Heavy cream (USDA)	1 cup	840	7
Unwhipped (USDA)	1 tbsp.	55	1
Heavy whipping (Meadow Gold)	1 tbsp.	50	.5
36% fat (Sealtest)	1 tbsp.	52	.5
Unwhipped (USDA)	1 cup (8.4 oz.) or 2 cups whipped	838	7.4
Light cream (USDA)	1 tbsp.	45	1
Coffee or table (USDA)	1 cup	505	10
(USDA)	1 tbsp.	30	1

J
M

Food and Description	Measure or Quantity	Calories	Carbohydrates (grams)
Light, table, or coffee,			
16% fat *(Sealtest)*	1 tbsp.	26	.6
18% fat *(Sealtest)*	1 tbsp.	28	.6
25% fat *(Sealtest)*	1 tbsp.	37	.5
Light, whipping, 30% fat			
(Sealtest)	1 tbsp.	44	.5
Sour cream *(USDA)*	1 cup	485	10
(USDA)	1 tbsp.	25	1
(Borden)	1 cup	454	7.7
	1 tbsp.	28	.4
(Breakstone)	8-oz. container	464	8.4
	1 tbsp.	29	.6
(Breakstone)	2 tbsp.	58	3.7
(Sealtest)	1 tbsp.	28	.5
Half & Half *(Sealtest)*	1 tbsp.	20	.5
Imitation *(Royal Danish--Beatrice Foods)*	1 oz.	60	2
Imitation, non-dairy *(Sealtest)*	1 tbsp.	30	1.1
Imitation, Sour treat *(Delite)*	1 tbsp.	25	.8
Imitation, Zest, 13.5% vegetable fat *(Borden)*	1 tbsp.	24	.9
Dried *(Data from General Mills)*	1 oz.	188	8.0
Sour dairy dressing *(Sealtest)*	1 tbsp.	22	.7
Sour dressing, Imitation sour cream made with nonfat dry milk *(USDA)*	1 tbsp.	20	1
	1 cup	440	17.0
Cultured *(Breakstone)*	2 tbsp.	54	4.6
Dry, whole, packed *(USDA)*	1 cup (5.1 oz.)	728	55.4
Spooned *(USDA)*	1 cup (4.3 oz.)	607	46.2

Food and Description	Measure or Quantity	Calories	Carbohydrates (grams)
Nonfat, instant, low density (1-1/3 cups needed for reconstitution to 1 qt.) (USDA)	1 cup	245	35
Nonfat, instant, high density (7/8 cup needed for reconstitution to 1 qt.) (USDA)	1 cup	375	54
Nonfat, instant (Carnation)	1 cup (2.4 oz.)	244	37.4
*(Carnation)	1 cup (8.6 oz.)	81	12.4
Nonfat, instant, chocolate (Carnation)	1 cup (2.4 oz.)	260	44.1
*(Carnation)	1 cup (8.6 oz.)	129	21.9
Nonfat, instant *(Pet)	1 cup	81	11.8
*(Sanalac)	1 cup	82	11.6
*(Weight Watchers)	1 packet (3 grams)	10	1.4
Evaporated, Canned, Regular (Borden)	14.5-oz. can	563	39.9
(Carnation)	1 cup (8.9 oz.)	348	25.0
(Pet)	1 cup	352	24.0
Skimmed (Carnation)	1 cup (9 oz.)	192	27.9
Goat, Whole (USDA)	1 cup	163	11.2
Human (USDA)	1 oz. (by wt.)	22	2.7
Instant Breakfast (Carnation) Special Morning, chocolate.	1 pkg.	188	31.5
Special Morning, chocolate malt.	1 pkg.	188	31.1
Special Morning, strawberry.	1 pkg.	188	33.4

J
M

*Prepared as package directs.

Food and Description	Measure or Quantity	Cal-ories	Carbo-hydrates (grams)
Milk, Skim, Fresh, (Borden)	1 cup	99	13.6
(Sealtest)	1 cup	79	11.3
Diet (Sealtest)	1 cup	103	13.8
Light n'Lively, low fat (Sealtest)	1 cup	114	13.6
Lite-line, Fortified, low fat (Borden)	1 cup	119	14.2
Pro-line, 2% fat (Borden)	1 cup	140	14.2
Skim-line, Fortified (Borden)	1 cup	99	13.6
Vita Lure, 2% fat (Sealtest)	1 cup	137	13.6
Vitamin A & D (Meadow Gold)	1 cup	90	11
Nonfat (skim (USDA)	1 cup	90	12
Partly skimmed, 2% nonfat, Milk solids added (USDA)	1 cup	145	15
Milk, Whole, fresh, 3.25% fat, Homogenized (Borden)	1 cup	152	11.8
3.25% fat (Sealtest)	1 cup	144	10.8
3.5% fat (Sealtest)	1 cup	151	11.0
3.5% fat (USDA)	1 cup	160	12
3.7% fat (Sealtest)	1 cup	157	11.1
Multivitamin (Sealtest)	1 cup	151	11.0
Grade A, Pasteurized Homog-enized Vitamin D Milk (Meadow Gold)	1 cup	150	12
Milk Beverages, Cocoa, homemade (USDA)	1 cup	245	27
Cocoa mix, hot (Hershey)	1 oz.	110	20
(Nestle's)	1-oz. pkg.	101	22.1
Cocoa mix *(Kraft)	1 cup	129	26.5
(Kraft)	1 oz.	105	21.3
Cocoa mix, Ever Ready (Nestle's)	3 heap. tsp.	105	19.6
Cocoa mix, without nonfat dry milk (USDA)	1 oz.	98	25.3
Cocoa mix, with nonfat dry milk (USDA)	1 oz.	102	20.1
Cocoa, instant (Hershey's)	1 oz.	110	24

*Prepared as package directs.

Food and Description	Measure or Quantity	Cal-ories	Carbo-hydrates (grams)
Special Morning, vanilla.	1 pkg.	188	33.4
Butterscotch.	1 pkg.	128	24.4
Chocolate.	1 pkg.	128	22.6
Chocolate fudge.	1 pkg.	128	22.2
Chocolate malt.	1 pkg.	128	21.7
Chocolate marshmallow	1 pkg.	128	22.8
Coffee.	1 pkg.	128	24.2
Eggnog.	1 pkg.	128	23.5
Chocolate malt (Pillsbury)	1 oz.	101	18.8
Strawberry (Pillsbury)	1 oz.	104	19.2
Vanilla (Pillsbury)	1 oz.	101	17.9
Instant Breakfast Mix,			
Chocolate (Pillsbury)	1 pouch + 8 oz. milk	290	38
Strawberry (Pillsbury)	1 pouch + 8 oz. milk	290	39
Malted Milk, Dry powder, approx. 3 heaping teaspoons per oz.			
(USDA)	1 oz.	115	20
Dry powder *(USDA)	1 cup	245	28
Malted Milk Mix, Chocolate,			
Instant (Borden)	2 heap. tsp.	77	16.0
Chocolate (Carnation)	3 heap. tsp.	85	18.3
Chocolate, dry (Kraft)	2 heap. tsp.	51	10.0
Chocolate *(Kraft)	1 cup	241	29.8
Natural, Instant (Borden)	2 heap. tsp.	80	13.4
Natural (Carnation)	3 heap. tsp.	88	15.6
Natural, dry (Kraft)	2 heap. tsp.	52	92
Natural *(Kraft)	1 cup (8.6 oz.)	240	27.7
Powder (Horlicks)	1 oz.	118	19.8
Tablet (Horlicks)	1 tablet	6	.9
Milk, Lowfat, 1% milkfat,			
Vitamin A & D (Meadow Gold)	1 cup	100	11
2% milkfat, Grade A, Vitamin A & D, Viva (Meadow Gold)	1 cup	130	13

J
M

*Prepared as package directs.

Food and Description	Measure or Quantity	Calories	Carbo-hydrates (grams)
Cocoa mix, instant (Swiss Miss)	1 oz.	106	20.4
Cocoa mix, instant, chocolate marshmallow (Carnation)	1 pkg. (1 oz.)	112	21.0
Cocoa mix, instant, milk chocolate (Carnation)	1 pkg. (1 oz.)	120	20.5
Cocoa mix, instant, rich chocolate (Carnation)	1 pkg. (1 oz.)	109	20.4
Sweetened, fudge (USDA)	1 tbsp.	63	10.3
Thin type (USDA)	1 tbsp.	47	11.9
(Hershey's)	1 tbsp.	69	16.7
(Smucker's)	1 tbsp.	47	11.6
Low calorie, chocotop (Slim-ette)	1 tbsp.	9	1.6
(Tillie Lewis)	1 tbsp.	4	.6
Reindeer (USDA)	1 oz. (by wt.)	66	1.2
YOGHURT			
Apricot (Breakstone)	8-oz. container	220	37.4
(Dannon)	8-oz. container	258	51.1
Swiss Parfait (Breakstone)	8-oz. container	249	42.9
Blueberry (Breakstone)	8-oz. container	252	46.3
(Meadow Gold)	8-oz. container	249	54.0
Light n' Lively (Sealtest)	8-oz. container	257	50.6
(Sugar-Lo)	8-oz. container	117	14.6
Swiss Parfait (Breakstone)	8-oz. container	286	53.1

Food and Description	Measure or Quantity	Cal-ories	Carbo-hydrates (grams)
Swiss Style *(Meadow Gold)*	8-oz. container	245	49.0
Boysenberry *(Dannon)*	8-oz. container	258	51.1
(Meadow Gold)	8-oz. container	249	54.0
Cherry *(Dannon)*	8-oz. container	258	51.1
(Meadow Gold)	8-oz. container	249	54.0
Dark *(Sugar-Lo)*	8-oz. container	117	14.6
Cinnamon Apple *(Breakstone)*	8-oz. container	229	39.9
Coffee *(Dannon)*	8-oz. container	198	33.3
Cuplet, Any flavor, Danny *(Dannon)*	4-oz. container	198	33.3
Dutch Apple *(Dannon)*	8-oz. container	258	51.1
Flavored *(Dannon)*	8 oz.	200	32
Stay 'n Shape, Vanilla *(Breakstone)*	8 oz.	205	14.8
Stay 'n Shape, Strawberry *(Breakstone)*	8 oz.	245	20.6
Fruit *(Dannon)*	8 oz.	260	49
Strawberry, Lowfat, Swiss style *(Viva)*	1 cup	250	47
Frozen pop, Danny *(Dannon)*	2½-oz. pop	127	18.0
Honey, Swiss Parfait *(Breakstone)*	8-oz. container	277	51.5
Lemon, Light n' Lively *(Sealtest)*	8-oz. container	229	43.4
Swiss Parfait *(Breakstone)*	8-oz. container	254	44.9

J
M

Food and Description	Measure or Quantity	Calories	Carbohydrates (grams)
Lime, Swiss Parfait *(Breakstone)*	8-oz. container	243	40.1
Mandarin Orange, Swiss Parfait *(Breakstone)*	8-oz. container	263	48.3
Mandarin Orange, Swiss Style *(Borden)*	5-oz. container	142	28.7
(Borden)	8-oz. container	227	45.9
Parfait, Black Cherry *(Breakstone)*	8 oz.	256	19.8
Peach *(Breakstone)*	8 oz.	254	20.9
Strawberry *(Breakstone)*	8 oz.	260	22.3
Peach *(Meadow Gold)*	8 oz. container	249	54.0
(Sugar-Lo)	8-oz. container	117	14.6
Melba, Swiss Parfait *(Breakstone)*	8-oz. container	268	49.4
Swiss Style *(Borden)*	5-oz. container	138	27.8
(Borden)	8-oz. container	221	44.5
Pineapple *(Breakstone)*	8-oz. container	220	37.9
(Meadow Gold)	8-oz. container	249	54.0
Light n' Lively *(Sealtest)*	8-oz. container	241	47.2
(Sugar-Lo)	8-oz. container	117	14.8
Pineapple-orange *(Dannon)*	8-oz. container	258	51.1

Food and Description	Measure or Quantity	Calories	Carbohydrates (grams)
Plain (Breakstone)	8-oz. container	141	12.7
Plain or vanilla, Made from partially skimmed milk (USDA)	½ cup	61	6.3
(USDA)	8-oz. container	113	11.8
Plain (Dannon)	8 oz.	150	17
Stay 'n Shape (Breakstone)	8 oz.	145	7.1
Swiss Style (Borden)	5-oz. container	82	9.9
(Borden)	8-oz. container	131	15.9
Prune whip (Breakstone)	8-oz. container	231	41.1
(Dannon)	8-oz. container	258	51.1
Soft, Frozen (Danny-Yo)	3½-oz.	115	21
Strawberry, Swiss Style (Borden)	5-oz. container	142	27.8
Swiss Style (Borden)	8-oz. container	227	44.5
(Dannon)	8-oz. container	258	51.1
(Meadow Gold)	8-oz. container	249	54.0
Swiss Miss (Sanna)	4-oz. container	125	19.0
Light n' Lively (Sealtest)	8-oz. container	234	44.3
(Sugar-Lo)	8-oz. container	111	13.2
Raspberry, Swiss Style (Borden)	5-oz. container	147	29.5
Swiss Style (Borden)	8-oz. container	236	47.2

Food and Description	Measure or Quantity	Calories	Carbo-hydrates (grams)
(Breakstone)	8-oz. container	249	45.8
Red, Swiss Parfait (Breakstone)	8-oz. container	263	46.5
(Dannon)	8-oz. container	258	51.1
Swiss Style (Meadow Gold)	8-oz. container	245	49.0
Swiss Miss (Sanna)	4-oz. container	125	19.0
Red, Light n' Lively (Sealtest)	8-oz. container	225	41.8
(Sugar-Lo)	8-oz. container	118	14.8
Vanilla, Swiss Style (Borden)	5-oz. container	148	28.4
Swiss Style (Borden) 8-oz.	5-oz. container	235	45.4
(Dannon)	8-oz. container	198	33.3
Yoghurt, Viva, Swiss style, plain, lowfat (Meadow Gold)	1 cup	180	23
	8-oz. container	245	49.0
Yoghurt, Made from whole milk (USDA)	1 cup	150	12
Yoghurt, Made from partially skimmed milk (USDA)	1 cup	125	13

NUTS

Food and Description	Measure or Quantity	Calories	Carbo-hydrates (grams)
Almonds, Shelled, whole kernels (USDA)	1 cup	850	28
Dry roasted (Planters)	1 oz.	170	5
Chopped (USDA)	1 cup	759	24.8

Food and Description	Measure or Quantity	Calories	Carbo-hydrates (grams)
Chopped (*Blue Diamond*)	1 cup	1008	38.7
Blanched, salted (*USDA*)	1 cup	984	30.6
Almonds, Flavored, Barbecue, cheese, French-fried, onion-garlic or smokehouse style	1 oz.	180	9.5
Almonds, Roasted, Dry, Salted (*Planters*)	1 oz.	191	5.5
Brazil Nut, Whole (*USDA*)	1 cup (14 nuts, 4.3 oz. with shell)	383	6.4
Shelled (*USDA*)	½ cup (2.5 oz.)	458	7.6
Cashew nuts, Roasted (*USDA*)	1 cup	785	41
Roasted (*Planters*)	1 oz.	170	8
Dry roasted (*Planters*)	1 oz.	160	8
Dry Roasted (*Skippy*)	1 oz.	165	8.0
Chestnut, Fresh, Shelled (*USDA*)	4 oz.	220	47.7
Coconut, fresh meat only, Piece approx. 2× 2 × ½ in. (*USDA*)	1 piece	155	4
Shredded or grated, firmly packed (*USDA*)	1 cup	450	12
Macadamia, Shelled (*USDA*)	4 oz.	784	18.0
Mixed nuts, Dry roasted (*Planters*)	1 oz.	160	6
Dry roasted (*Skippy*)	1 oz.	170	5.4
Regular (*Planters*)	1 oz.	180	6
Peanuts, Roasted, salted, halves (*USDA*)	1 cup	840	27
Dry roasted (*Planters*)	1 oz.	160	5
Dry roasted (*Skippy*)	1 oz.	165	4.1
Old fashioned (*Planters*)	1 oz.	170	5
Peanut butter (*USDA*)	1 tbsp.	95	3
Smooth (*Peter Pan*)	2 tbsp.	190	6
(*Planters*)	1 oz.	190	6
Creamy (*Skippy*)	1 tbsp.	95	2

N P

171

Food and Description	Measure or Quantity	Calories	Carbohydrates (grams)
(S & W)	1 tbsp.	93	2
Low sodium, smooth *(Peter Pan)*	2 tbsp.	190	4
Super chunk *(Skippy)*	1 tbsp.	95	1.9
Pecans, In shell *(USDA)*	1 lb. (weighed in shell)	1652	35.1
Shelled, Whole *(USDA)*	1 lb.	3116	66.2
Halves *(USDA)*	1 cup	740	16
	½ cup	371	7.9
	12-14 halves	96	2.0
Dry roasted *(Planters)*	1-oz.	190	5
Shelled, chopped *(USDA)*	½ cup	357	7.6
	1 tbsp.	48	1.0
Pine Nut, Pignolias, shelled *(USDA)*	4 oz.	626	13.2
Pistachios, In shell *(USDA)*	4 oz. (weighed in shell)	337	10.8
	½ cup	197	6.3
Shelled *(USDA)*	½ cup	368	11.8
	1 tbsp.	46	1.5
Dry roasted *(Planters)*	1 oz.	170	5
Sunflower nuts, Dry roasted *(Planters)*	1 oz.	160	5
Walnuts, Black, in shell, whole *(USDA)*	1 lb. (weighed in shell)	627	14.8
Black, shelled, whole *(USDA)*	4 oz.	712	16.8
Black, chopped *(USDA)*	1 cup	790	19
English or Persian, In shell, whole *(USDA)*	1 lb. (weighed in shell)	1329	32.2
English or Persian, Shelled, whole *(USDA)*	4 oz.	738	17.9

Food and Description	Measure or Quantity	Calories	Carbohydrates (grams)
English or Persian, Chopped (USDA)	½ cup	391	9.5
	1 tbsp.	49	1.2
English or Persian, Halves (USDA)	½ cup	326	7.9
English or Persian (Diamond)	¾ cup	564	15.0
	15 halves	99	2.7

PANCAKES AND WAFFLES

Food and Description	Measure or Quantity	Calories	Carbohydrates (grams)
Pancakes, 4 in. diam., wheat enriched flour, home recipe (USDA)	1 cake	60	9
Blueberry pancake mix (Hungry Jack)	3 pancakes 4 in. diam.	340	43
Buckwheat pancake & waffle mix (Aunt Jemima)	3 pancakes 4 in. diam.	183	22.5
Buckwheat pancakes, made from mix with egg & milk (USDA)	1 cake	55	6
Plain or buttermilk, made from mix with egg & milk (USDA)	1 cake	60	9
Buttermilk pancake mix (Hungry Jack)	3 pancakes 4 in. diam.	240	29
Buttermilk pancake & waffle mix (Aunt Jemima)	3 pancakes 4 in. diam.	251	33.7
Pancake & waffle mix (Aunt Jemima Original)	3 pancakes	181	23.5
Pancake & link sausage breakfast, frozen (Swanson)	1 breakfast	500	50
Waffles, with enriched flour, 7 in. diam. (USDA)	1 waffle	210	28
Made with mix, enriched, egg & milk added, 7 in. diam. (USDA)	1 waffle	205	27

N
P

Food and Description	Measure or Quantity	Calories	Carbohydrates (grams)
Frozen (*Aunt Jemima*)	2 waffle sections	114	15.7
Frozen (*Eggo*)	1 waffle	120	17
With imitation blueberries, frozen (*Eggo*)	1 waffle	130	17

PIES AND PASTRY, FILLINGS, CRUSTS

Food and Description	Measure or Quantity	Calories	Carbohydrates (grams)
Apple Turnover (*Pillsbury*)	1 turnover	170	26
Blueberry Turnover, Frozen (*Pepperidge Farm*)	1 turnover (3.3 oz.)	321	32.0
Cherry Turnover (*Pillsbury*)	1 turnover	180	25
Danish pastry, plain, (without fruit or nuts) round piece approx. 4¼ in. diam. by 1 in. (*USDA*)	1 pastry	275	30
Plain (*USDA*)	1 oz.	120	13
Doughnuts, Cake type (*USDA*)	1 doughnut	125	16
Chocolate iced doughnuts, frozen (*Morton*)	1.5 oz.	150	19
Jelly donuts, frozen (*Morton*)	1.83 oz.	180	22
Plain cake donuts (*Morton*)	1.71 oz.	170	23
Powdered cake donut, frozen (*Morton*)	1.87 oz.	190	28
Apple filling, Canned, sweetened (*Comstock*)	½ cup	178	45.6
Canned, sweetened (*Lucky Leaf*)	8 oz.	248	60.8
Canned, sweetened (*Musselman's*)	1 cup	283	
Canned, unsweetened (*Lucky Leaf*)	8 oz.	98	23.2
French Apple filling, Canned, sweetened (*Comstock*)	½ cup	97	41.7
Bavarian Pie Filling, Canned (*Lucky Leaf*)	8 oz.	306	51.8
Blackberry filling, Canned (*Comstock*)	1 cup	438	108.5

Food and Description	Measure or Quantity	Calories	Carbohydrates (grams)
Canned (Lucky Leaf)	8 oz.	258	62.4
Blueberry filling, Canned			
(Comstock)	1 cup	332	82.8
Canned (Lucky Leaf)	8 oz.	256	61.4
Canned (Musselman's)	1 cup	321	
Butterscotch filling, Regular,			
sweetened *(Royal)	½ cup	191	31.8
Sweetened, regular			
*(My-T-Fine)	½ cup	175	32.5
Low-calorie *(D-Zerta)	½ cup	107	4.8
Cherry filling (Comstock)	1 cup	334	84.6
(Lucky Leaf)	8 oz.	242	58.2
(Musselman's)	1 cup	400	
Chocolate filling, Sweetened,			
Regular, Dark 'N' Sweet			
*(Royal)	½ cup	194	30.5
Sweetened, regular,			
Fudge *(Jello)	½ cup	174	29.5
Sweetened, Regular, Milk			
Chocolate *(Jello)	½ cup	174	29.5
Coconut filling, Toasted,			
Instant *(Royal)	½ cup	186	28.4
Cream, instant *(Jello)	½ cup	188	29.0
Cream, regular *(Jello)	½ cup	175	25.8
Lemon filling, Canned			
(Comstock)	½ cup	174	44.0
Canned (Lucky Leaf)	8 oz.	412	95.4
Mincemeat filling			
(Crosse & Blackwell)	½ cup	480	114.4
(Comstock)	½ cup	209	48.0
Ready-to-use (None Such)	½ cup	327	75.8
With brandy & rum			
(None Such)	½ cup	305	66.2
Peach filling (Musselman's)	1 cup	292	
(Lucky Leaf)	8 oz.	300	74.0
(Comstock)	½ cup	175	47.1

*Prepared as package directs.

N
P

Food and Description	Measure or Quantity	Calories	Carbohydrates (grams)
Pumpkin filling, Canned			
Del Monte)	1 cup	218	61.2
Canned (Comstock)	1 cup	366	90.2
Pie Crust, Baked shell made			
with enriched flour (USDA)	1 shell	900	79
Mix including stick form, 10-oz. pkg. for double crust (USDA)	1 pkg.	1480	141
Mix (Betty Crocker)	1/16 pkg.	120	10
Mix (Flako)	1/6 of single 9-in. pie	116	11.7
Mix (Pillsbury)	1/6 of a 2-crust pie	290	27
Home recipe, Baked 9-in. pie (USDA)	1 crust	900	78.8
Frozen (Mrs. Smith's)	8-in. shell	760	62.4
(Mrs. Smith's)	Old fashioned 9-in. shell	1100	90.7
(Mrs. Smith's)	10-in. shell	1240	102.1
Mix, Dry, pkg. or stick (USDA)	10-oz. pkg. (2 crusts)	1482	140.6
Dry, pkg. or stick, prepared with water, baked *(USDA)	4 oz.	526	49.9
Dry, pkg. or stick, Double crust *(Betty Crocker)	1/6 of 2 crusts	302	24.1
Dry, pkg. or stick, Graham cracker *(Betty Crocker)	1/6 of crust	159	22.3
Dry, pkg. or stick *(Flako)	1/6 of 9-in. shell	121	12.0
Apple Pie (USDA)	1 sector	350	51
(Hostess)	1 pie	420	52
(Drake's)	2-oz. pie	200	25.2
(Tastykake)	4-oz. pie	380	58.6
Frozen (Banquet)	20 oz.	1440	213.2

*Prepared as package directs.

176

Food and Description	Measure or Quantity	Calories	Carbohydrates (grams)
	5-oz. serving	351	49.5
Frozen (Morton)	1/6 of 20-oz. pie	240	33.7
24-oz., Frozen (Morton)	4 oz.	300	43
Frozen (Mrs. Smith's)	1/6 of 8-in. pie	303	42.0
Frozen, Old fashion (Mrs. Smith's)	1/6 of 9-in. pie	508	74.6
Frozen, Dutch Apple (Mrs. Smith's)	1/6 of 8-in. pie	326	47.2
Apple Crumb, Frozen (Mrs. Smith's)	1/8 of 10-in. pie	429	62.4
Frozen, tart (Mrs. Smith's)	1/6 of 8-in. pie	266	44.0
French Apple (Tastykake)	4½-oz. pie	451	64.3
Banana Pie, Cream or Custard, Home recipe (USDA)	1/6 of 9-in. pie (5.4 oz.)	336	46.7
(Tastykake)	4-oz. pie	485	82.4
Frozen (Mrs. Smith's)	1/6 of 8-in. pie (2.3 oz.)	203	23.2
Banana Cream Pie, frozen (Banquet)	14 oz.	1032	119.6
	2½-oz. serving	185	25.0
Frozen (Morton)	2.66 oz.	200	26
Blackberry, Home recipe, 2 crust (USDA)	1/6 of 9-in. pie	384	54.4
(Tastykake)	4-oz. pie	386	60.1

*Prepared as package directs.

177

Food and Description	Measure or Quantity	Calories	Carbohydrates (grams)
Frozen *(Banquet)*	5-oz. serving	376	55.5
Blueberry, Home recipe, 2 crust *(USDA)*	1/6 of 9-in. pie	382	55.1
Frozen *(Banquet)*	20 oz.	1520	225.1
	5-oz. serving	366	55.8
(Hostess)	1 pie	410	52
24-oz., frozen *(Morton)*	4 oz.	300	42
Frozen *(Mrs. Smith's)*	1/6 of 8-in. pie	288	39.2
Frozen, Golden deluxe *(Mrs. Smith's)*	1/8 of 10-in. pie	379	51.4
Butterscotch, Home recipe *(USDA)*	1/6 of 9-in. pie	406	58.2
Frozen, Cream *(Banquet)*	2½-oz. serving	187	27.0
Cheese, Frozen, pineapple *(Mrs. Smith's)*	1/8 of 8-in. pie (4 oz.)	273	36.4
Frozen, pineapple *(Mrs. Smith's)*	1/8 of 10-in. pie (5.4 oz.)	341	45.4
Cherry, Frozen, Golden deluxe *(Mrs. Smith's)*	1/8 of 10-in. pie	361	46.4
Frozen *(Mrs. Smith's)*	1/6 of 8-in. pie	274	35.4
Frozen, 24 oz. *(Morton)*	4 oz.	300	42
Frozen *(Morton)*	1/6 of 20-oz. pie	250	35.7
Frozen *(Banquet)*	20 oz.	1366	203
	5 oz.	352	50.2

Food and Description	Measure or Quantity	Calories	Carbohydrates (grams)
(Hostess)	1 pie 4½ oz.	337	56.0
(Drake's)	2-oz. pie	201	25.4
2 crust (USDA)	1 sector	350	52
Chocolate, Frozen, cream, velvet nut (Kraft)	1/6 of 16-¾ oz. pie	303	30.4
Frozen, cream, tart (Pepperidge Farm)	1 tart (3 oz.)	306	35.2
Frozen, Cream (Mrs. Smith's)	1/6 of 8-in. pie	224	25.5
Nut (Tastykake)	4½-oz. pie	451	64.3
Meringue, Home recipe (USDA)	6 of 9-in. pie	353	46.9
Chiffon, Home recipe (USDA)	1/6 of 9-in. pie	459	61.2
Chocolate cream pie, 16 oz., frozen (Morton)	2.66 oz.	220	29
Chocolate cream pie, frozen (Banquet)	14 oz.	1064	131
	2½-oz. serving	202	28.5
Coconut, Custard, Frozen (Mrs. Smith's)	1/6 of 8-in. pie	272	31.7
(Mrs. Smith's)	1/8 of 10-in. pie	344	39.7
Cream (Tastykake)	4-oz. pie	467	48.4
Cream, Frozen (Banquet)	2½-oz. serving	209	24.2
Cream, Frozen (Morton)	¼ of 14.4-oz. pie	278	37.1
Cream, Frozen (Mrs. Smith's)	1/6 of 8-in. pie	212	24.5
Cream Frozen, Tart (Pepperidge Farm)	3-oz. tart	310	29.0

N
P

179

Food and Description	Measure or Quantity	Calories	Carbohydrates (grams)
Custard, Frozen *(Banquet)*	5-oz. serving	294	39.8
Custard, Frozen *(Morton)*	1/6 of 20-oz. pie	203	27.7
(Morton)	1/8 of 46-oz. pie	506	60.3
Coconut-Custard, Home recipe *(USDA)*	1/6 of 9-in. pie	357	37.8
Custard pie, frozen *(Banquet)*	20 oz.	1236	190.5
	5 oz.	274	41.2
Home recipe *(USDA)*	1/6 of 9-in. pie	331	35.6
Custard pie, 1 crust *(USDA)*	1 sector	285	30
Lemon Tart, Frozen *(Pepperidge Farm)*	1 tart	317	36.4
Chiffon, Home recipe *(USDA)*	1/6 of 9-in. pie	338	47.3
(Hostess)	1 pie	450	56
Meringue, Frozen *(Mrs. Smith's)*	1/6 of 8-in. pie	288	41.1
Lemon meringue pie, 1 crust *(USDA)*	1 sector	305	45
Lemon Cream, Frozen *(Mrs. Smith's)*	1/6 of 8-in. pie	203	22.7
Frozen *(Morton)*	¼ of 14.4-oz. pie	262	36.4
Frozen *(Banquet)*	14 oz.	1008	131
	2½-oz. serving	179	25.5
Lime Pie Filling, Mix, Key Lime *(Royal)*	1/8 of pie (inc. crust, 4.2 oz.)	301	43.4

Food and Description	Measure or Quantity	Calories	Carbohydrates (grams)
Lime Pie, Key lime, Cream, Frozen *(Banquet)*	2½-oz. serving	204	27.5
Mince, Frozen *(Mrs. Smith's)*	1/6 of 8-in. pie	335	48.2
(Mrs. Smith's)	1/8 of 10-in. pie	456	63.4
Frozen *(Morton)*	1/6 of 20-in. pie	247	35.8
(Tastykake)	4-oz. pie	373	50.8
2 crust *(USDA)*	1 sector	365	56
Mincemeat pie, Frozen *(Banquet)*	20 oz.	1514	230.8
	5-oz. serving	401	62.8
Peach, Frozen *(Mrs. Smith's)*	1/6 of 8-in. pie	299	42.0
(Mrs. Smith's)	1/6 of 9-in. pie	506	73.7
(Mrs. Smith's)	1/8 of 10-in. pie	394	55.3
24 oz., Frozen *(Morton)*	4 oz.	290	40
Frozen *(Morton)*	1/6 of 20-oz. pie	245	34.9
Frozen *(Banquet)*	20 oz.	1315	179.2
	5-oz. serving	320	45.5
(Hostess)	1 pie	450	51
Home recipe, 2 crust *(USDA)*	1/6 of 9-in. pie	403	60.4
Pumpkin pie mix, plain *(Libby's)*	1/6 of 9-in. baked pie	330	49
Frozen *(Mrs. Smith's)*	1/6 of 8-in. pie	229	33.6
(Mrs. Smith's)	1/8 of 10-in. pie	296	43.2

N
P

Food and Description	Measure or Quantity	Calories	Carbohydrates (grams)
24 oz., Frozen (Morton)	4 oz.	240	35
(Morton)	1/6 of 20-oz. pie	167	26.2
(Morton)	1/8 of 46-oz. pie.	488	61.1
Frozen (Banquet)	20 oz.	1236	193.9
	5-oz. serving	306	46.5
(Tastykake)	4-oz. pie	368	50.5
1 crust (USDA)	1 sector	275	32
Toast-R-Cakes, Blueberry, fresh or frozen (S.B. Thomas)	1 cake	110	17.4
Bran, fresh or frozen (S. B. Thomas)	1 cake	115	19.6
Corn, fresh or frozen (S. B. Thomas)	1 cake	120	18.8
Orange (Thomas)	1 piece	117	17.9
Toastee, Blueberry (Howard Johnson's)	1 piece	121	17.0
Cinnamon raisin (Howard Johnson's)	1 piece	114	17.3
Corn (Howard Johnson's)	1 piece	112	18.2
Orange (Howard Johnson's)	1 piece	113	15.5
Pound (Howard Johnson's)	1 piece	111	15.9
Toastette, Apple (Nabisco)	1 piece	184	32.3
Blueberry (Nabisco)	1 piece	184	33.0
Brown sugar, cinnamon (Nabisco)	1 piece	189	31.9
Cherry (Nabisco)	1 piece	182	32.7
Orange marmalade (Nabisco)	1 piece	181	32.1
Peach (Nabisco)	1 piece	183	32.7
Strawberry (Nabisco)	1 piece	184	32.7
Corn Treats (Arnold)	1.1-oz. piece	111	17.1

Food and Description	Measure or Quantity	Calories	Carbo-hydrates (grams)
POULTRY			
Capon, Raw, ready to cook (USDA)	1 lb. (weighed with bones)	937	0
Raw, Meat with skin (USDA)	4 oz.	330	0
Capon Giblets, Raw.	2 oz.	125	.2
Fryer, raw.	2 oz.	58	<.1
Roaster, raw.	2 oz.	77	1.0
Chicken, Fried, ½ breast, flesh and skin only (USDA)	2.7 oz.	155	1
Fried, ½ breast, with bone (USDA)	3.3 oz.	155	1
Chicken, Drumstick fried, with bone (USDA)	2.1 oz.	90	Trace
Drumstick fried, flesh and skin only (USDA)	1.3 oz.	90	Trace
Chicken, Broiler, cooked, meat only (USDA)	4 oz.	154	0
Chicken, canned, boneless (USDA)	3 oz.	170	0
Boned chicken with broth (Swanson)	2½ oz.	110	1
Chicken & Dumplings (Swanson)	7½ oz.	230	18
Chicken à la King (Swanson)	5¼ oz.	190	9
Chicken Stew, Canned (Swanson)	7½ oz.	180	18
Chicken Cacciatore, Canned (Hormel)	1-lb. can	386	8.2
Chicken, cooked, flesh only, broiled (USDA)	3 oz.	115	0
Chicken, Roasted, light meat, without skin (USDA)	4 oz.	206	0
Dark meat, without skin (USDA)	4 oz.	209	0
Chicken, Stewed, dark meat without skin (USDA)	4 oz.	235	0

N
P

Food and Description	Measure or Quantity	Calories	Carbohydrates (grams)
Light meat, without skin (USDA)	4 oz.	204	0
Chicken Spread, Canned (Swanson)	1 oz.	70	2
Duck, Raw, domesticated, ready-to-cook (USDA)	1 lb. (weighed with bones)	1213	0
Raw, domesticated, ready-to-cook, meat & skin (USDA)	4 oz.	370	0
Raw, Domesticated, Ready-to-cook, Meat only (USDA)	4 oz.	187	0
Wild, raw, dressed (USDA)	1 lb. (weighed dressed)	613	0
Wild, raw, dressed, meat, skin & giblets (USDA)	4 oz.	264	0
Wild, raw, dressed, meat only (USDA)	4 oz.	156	0
Goose, Domesticated, raw, ready-to-cook (USDA)	1 lb. (weighed with bones)	1172	0
Domesticated, raw, total edible (USDA)	4 oz.	401	0
Domesticated, roasted, total edible (USDA)	4 oz.	483	0
Domesticated, roasted, meat only (USDA)	4 oz.	264	0
Pheasant, Raw, Ready-to-cook (USDA)	1 lb. (weighed with bones)	596	0
Raw, ready-to-cook, meat & skin (USDA)	4 oz.	172	0
Raw, ready-to-cook, meat only (USDA)	4 oz.	184	0
Raw, ready-to-cook, giblets (USDA)	2 oz.	79	.9

Food and Description	Measure or Quantity	Cal- ories	Carbo- hydrates (grams)
Squab, Pigeon, raw, dressed (USDA)	1 lb. (weighed with feet, inedible viscera & bones)	569	0
Meat & skin, raw (USDA)	4 oz.	333	0
Meat only, raw (USDA)	4 oz.	161	0
Light meat only, raw, without skin (USDA)	4 oz.	142	0
Giblets, raw (USDA)	1 oz.	44	.3
Turkey, 1 slice white, 4 in. long, 2 in. wide, ¼ in. thick and 2 slices dark, 2½ in. long, 1-5/8 in. wide, ¼ in. thick (USDA)	3 oz.	162	0
Boned turkey with broth, canned (Swanson)	2½ oz.	110	0

SALAD DRESSINGS AND MIXES

Food and Description	Measure or Quantity	Cal- ories	Carbo- hydrates (grams)
Salad Dressings (Bennett's)	1 tbsp.	50	2
Regular & low calorie, Bacon (Lawry's)	1 pkg.	69	11.9
Salad Dressings, Blue cheese dressings, (USDA)	1 tbsp.	75	1
Bleu cheese, Imperial (Kraft)	1 tbsp.	68	.9
Bleu cheese, Refrigerated (Kraft)	1 tbsp.	74	.8
Regular & low calorie, Bleu or blue cheese *(Good Seasons)	1 tbsp.	89	1.3
Bleu or blue cheese, Thick, creamy *(Good Seasons)	1 tbsp.	96	.9
Bleu or blue cheese (Lawry's)	1 pkg.	79	4.5
Salad Dressings, Bleu cheese, Roka (Kraft) Chunky blue cheese	1 tbsp.	55	.8

* Prepared as package directs.

Food and Description	Measure or Quantity	Calories	Carbohydrates (grams)
(Wish-Bone)	1 tbsp.	70	1
Boiled, home recipe (USDA)	1 tbsp.	26	2.4
Dietetic or Low Calorie, Bleu or blue, Low fat, 6% fat (USDA)	1 tbsp.	12	.7
Dietetic or Low Calorie, Bleu or blue, Chunky (Frenchette)	1 tbsp.	22	1.7
Dietetic or Low Calorie, Bleu or blue (Kraft)	1 tbsp.	13	5
Dietetic or Low Calorie, Bleu or blue (Slim-ette)	1 tbsp.	12	.1
Caesar, Golden (Kraft)	1 tbsp.	63	.8
Dietetic or Low Calorie, Caesar (Frenchette)	1 tbsp.	33	1.6
Caesar (Lawry's)	1 tbsp.	70	.5
Regular or low calorie, Caesar garlic cheese (Lawry's)	1 pkg.	71	8.7
Salad Dressings, Caesar dressing (Wish-Bone)	1 tbsp.	80	1
Canadian (Lawry's)	1 tbsp.	72	.6
Dietetic or Low Calorie, Catalina (Kraft)	1 tbsp.	15	2.6
Dietetic or Low Calorie, Cheese (Tillie Lewis)	1 tbsp.	12	.2
Regular or low calorie, Cheese Garlic *(Good Seasons)	1 tbsp.	84	.8
Salad Dressings, Dietetic or Low Calorie, Chef Style (Kraft)	1 tbsp.	16	2.6
Dietetic or Low Calorie, Chef's (Slim-ette)	1 tbsp.	14	2
Dietetic or Low Calorie, Chef's (Tillie Lewis)	1 tbsp.	2	.4
Coleslaw (Kraft)	1 tbsp.	62	3.4
Dietetic or Low Calorie, Coleslaw (Kraft)	1 tbsp.	28	3.4

* Prepared as package directs.

Food and Description	Measure or Quantity	Calories	Carbohydrates (grams)
Dietetic or Low Calorie, French, low fat, 1% fat, with artificial sweetener (USDA)	1 tbsp.	2	.3
Low calorie, French style dressing (Diet)	1 tbsp.	25	3
Dietetic or Low Calorie, French (Bennett's)	1 tbsp.	21	3.1
Dietetic or Low Calorie, French (Frenchette)	1 tbsp.	10	2.6
Dietetic or Low Calorie, French (Kraft)	1 tbsp.	21	2.0
Dietetic or Low Calorie, French (Tillie Lewis)	1 tbsp.	3	.8
Dietetic or Low Calorie, French (Wish-Bone)	1 tbsp.	23	3.3
Regular or Low Calorie, French, old fashion *(Good Seasons)	1 tbsp.	83	.5
Salad Dressings, French, home recipe with corn oil (USDA)	1 tbsp.	101	6
Regular or low calorie, French, thick, creamy *(Good Seasons)	1 tbsp.	97	1.9
Salad Dressings, French dressing, regular (USDA)	1 tbsp.	65	3
French dressing (Bennett's)	1 tbsp.	55	2
Regular or low calorie, French, old fashion (Lawry's)	1 pkg.	72	16.8
French, Riviera *(Good Seasons)	1 tbsp.	90	2.4
Salad Dressings, French, Family (Hellmann's)	1 tbsp.	65	2.9
French (Kraft)	1 tbsp.	65	1.9
French, Casino (Kraft)	1 tbsp.	60	3.0
French, Catalina (Kraft)	1 tbsp.	60	3.5
French, Miracle (Kraft)	1 tbsp.	57	2.5
French (Lawry's)	1 tbsp.	60	1.8

*Prepared as package directs.

Food and Description	Measure or Quantity	Calories	Carbohydrates (grams)
French, San Francisco (Lawry's)	1 tbsp.	53	.8
French, Blue, refrigerated (Marzetti)	1 tbsp.	70	3.4
French, Country (Marzetti)	1 tbsp.	72	3.6
Deluxe French dressing (Wish-Bone)	1 tbsp.	60	2
French dressing, special dietary, low fat with artificial sweeteners (USDA)	1 tbsp.	Trace	Trace
Fruit (Kraft)	1 tbsp.	52	3.0
Garlic French dressing (Wish-Bone)	1 tbsp.	70	3
Regular or low calorie, Garlic *(Good Seasons)	1 tbsp.	84	.8
Salad Dressings, Dietetic or Low Calorie, gourmet (Frenchette)	1 tbsp.	21	2.2
Garlic, French, Old Homestead (Hellmann's)	1 tbsp.	68	3.3
Garlic, creamy, refrigerated (Marzetti)	1 tbsp.	88	1.7
Garlic, creamy (Wish-Bone)	1 tbsp.	76	.7
Dietetic or Low Calorie, Green Goddess (Frenchette)	1 tbsp.	21	1.4
Dietetic or Low Calorie, Green Goddess (Slim-ette)	1 tbsp.	12	.5
Regular or low calorie, Green Goddess (Lawry's)	1 pkg.	69	12.7
Salad Dressings, Green Goddess (Kraft)	1 tbsp.	75	.7
Green Goddess (Lawry's)	1 tbsp.	59	.7
Green Goddess (Wish-Bone)	1 tbsp.	68	1.2
Green Onion (Kraft)	1 tbsp.	71	1.0
Hawaiian (Lawry's)	1 tbsp.	77	5.8
Herb & Garlic (Kraft)	1 tbsp.	87	.5

* Prepared as package directs.

Food and Description	Measure or Quantity	Calories	Carbohydrates (grams)
Low calorie Italian dressing (Wish-Bone)	1 tbsp.	18	1
Dietetic or Low Calorie, Italian (Tillie Lewis)	1 tbsp.	1	.3
Dietetic or Low Calorie, Italian (Slim-ette)	1 tbsp.	6	.3
Dietetic or Low Calorie, Italian (Kraft)	1 tbsp.	10	.7
Dietetic or Lo- Calorie, Italianette (Frenchette)	1 tbsp.	7	1.5
Low calorie, Italian dressing (Diet)	1 tbsp.	7	1
Dietetic or Low Calorie, Italian (Bennett's)	1 tbsp.	7	.9
Dietetic or Low Calorie, Italian (USDA)	1 tbsp.	8	.4
Italian (USDA)	1 tbsp.	83	1.0
Italian, True (Hellmann's)	1 tbsp.	84	.8
Italian (Kraft)	1 tbsp.	88	.7
Italian (Lawry's)	1 tbsp.	80	.9
Italian, with cheese (Lawry's)	1 tbsp.	60	4.7
Italian, Creamy (Marzetti)	1 tbsp.	73	1.8
Italian dressing (Wish-Bone)	1 tbsp.	80	1
Regular or low calorie, Italian *(Good Seasons)	1 tbsp.	84	.8
Italian, Cheese *(Good Seasons)	1 tbsp.	89	1.3
Italian, Mild *(Good Seasons)	1 tbsp.	89	1.3
Italian, Thick, creamy *(Good Seasons)	1 tbsp.	94	1.0
Italian (Lawry's)	1 pkg.	44	9.6
Italian, Cheese (Lawry's)	1 pkg.	69	9.4
Low calorie, Italian *(Good Seasons)	1 tsp.	3	.7
Salad Dressings, Commercial Mayonnaise, special dietary, low calorie (USDA)	1 tbsp.	20	1

Prepared as package directs

S V

Food and Description	Measure or Quantity	Calories	Carbohydrates (grams)
Diet Mayo 7, Imitation mayonnaise (Bennett's)	1 tbsp.	25	2
Dietetic or Low Calorie, Imitation Mayonnaise, May-Lo-Naise (Tillie Lewis)	1 tbsp.	9	.1
Dietetic or Low Calorie, Imitation Mayonnaise, Mayonette Gold (Frenchette)	1 tbsp.	33	1.9
Mayonnaise (USDA)	1 tbsp.	100	Trace
Mayonnaise (Barna)	1 tbsp.	95	.3
Mayonnaise (Bennett's)	1 tbsp.	110	0
Real Mayonnaise (Hellmann's/Best Foods)	1 tbsp.	100	0
Mayonnaise (Kraft)	1 tbsp.	102	.1
Mayonnaise (Kraft) Salad Bowl	1 tbsp.	102	.2
Mayonnaise (Nalley's)	1 oz.	214	.9
Mayonnaise (Saffola)	1 tbsp.	92	2.9
Mayonnaise, Salt Free (Healthlife)	1 oz.	211	.6
Commercial, Mayonnaise-type dressing (USDA)	1 tbsp.	65	2
Mayonnaise-type (USDA)	1 tbsp.	65	2.2
Mayonnaise-type, Imitation (Healthlife)	1 tbsp.	61	.9
Mayonnaise-type, Miracle Whip (Kraft)	1 tbsp.	69	1.8
Mayonnaise-type, Oil & vinegar (Kraft)	1 tbsp.	65	.6
Onion, California (Wish-Bone)	1 tbsp.	76	1.0
Dietetic or Low Calorie, Diet Mayo 7 (Bennett's)	1 tbsp.	23	2.0
Mayonnaise-type, Onion, creamy (Wish-Bone)	1 tbsp.	70	.8
Mayonnaise-type, Potato salad (Marzetti)	1 tbsp.	62	2.9
Mayonnaise-type, Ranch Style (Marzetti)	1 tbsp.	66	5.3

Food and Description	Measure or Quantity	Calories	Carbo-hydrates (grams)
Red wine vinegar & oil (Lawry's)	1 tbsp.	61	4.8
Romano Caesar (Marzetti)	1 tbsp.	69	1.3
Roquefort (USDA)	1 tbsp.	76	1.1
Regular or low calorie, Onion *(Good Seasons)	1 tbsp.	84	.8
Salad Dressings, Roquefort, refrigerated (Kraft)	1 tbsp.	56	.8
Roquefort, refrigerated (Marzetti)	1 tbsp.	80	.7
Russian (USDA)	1 tbsp.	74	1.6
Russian (Kraft)	1 tbsp.	55	4.3
Russian, Creamy (Kraft)	1 tbsp.	68	2.1
Russian, Creamy (Marzetti)	1 tbsp.	75	2.1
Russian dressing (Wish-Bone)	1 tbsp.	60	7
Dietetic or Low Calorie, Russian (Wish-Bone)	1 tbsp.	24	4.7
Salad Bowl (Kraft)	1 tbsp.	53	2.2
Salad 'n Sandwich (Kraft)	1 tbsp.	53	2.8
Salad Secret (Kraft)	1 tbsp.	56	1.8
Sherry (Lawry's)	1 tbsp.	55	1.6
Slaw, Regular or refrigerated (Marzetti's)	1 tbsp.	73	3.2
Spin Blend salad dressing (Hellmann's)	1 tbsp.	60	3
Sweet & Sour (Kraft)	1 tbsp.	28	6.5
Tahitian Isle (Wish-Bone)	1 tbsp.	54	7.0
Thousand Island Dressing (USDA)	1 tbsp.	80	3
Regular or low calorie, Thousand Island, thick, creamy *(Good Seasons)	1 tbsp.	80	1.7
Salad Dressings, Dietetic or Low Calorie, Thousand Island (Frenchette)	1 tbsp.	22	3.0
Dietetic or Low Calorie, Thousand Island (Kraft)	1 tbsp.	28	2.3

*Prepared as package directs.

191

Food and Description	Measure or Quantity	Calories	Carbohydrates (grams)
Dietetic or Low Calorie, Thousand Island, whipped (Tillie Lewis)	1 tbsp.	10	.2
Dietetic or Low Calorie, Thousand Island (Wish-Bone)	1 tbsp.	25	2.6
Thousand Island dressing, low calorie (USDA)	1 tbsp.	27	2.3
Thousand Island (Best Foods)	1 tbsp.	60	2.8
Thousand Island (Kraft)	1 tbsp.	71	1.9
Thousand Island, pourable (Kraft)	1 tbsp.	56	2.3
Thousand Island (Lawry's)	1 tbsp.	69	2.3
Thousand Island, refrigerated (Marzetti)	1 tbsp.	71	2.2
Thousand Island dressing (Wish-Bone)	1 tbsp.	70	3

SANDWICH SPREADS

Food and Description	Measure or Quantity	Calories	Carbohydrates (grams)
Chicken Spread, Canned (Underwood)	1 oz.	63	1.1
Corned Beef Spread (Underwood)	1 oz.	55	Trace
	1 tbsp.	27	.1
Sandwich Spread (USDA)	1 tbsp.	57	2.4
Low Calorie (USDA)	1 tbsp.	17	1.2
(Bennett's)	1 tbsp.	45	4
(Best Foods)	1 tbsp.	60	2
(Hellmann's)	1 tbsp.	62	2.4
(Kraft)	1 oz.	105	5.6
(Nalley's)	1 oz.	100	7.0
(Oscar Mayer)	1 oz.	60	4.9
Salad Bowl (Kraft)	1 oz.	101	5.7
Chicken Salad (Carnation)	1/5 can	99	4.2
Corned Beef (Carnation)	1/5 can	96	3.7
Ham & Cheese (Carnation)	1/5 can	80	4.0
Ham Salad (Carnation)	1/5 can	90	4.2
Pimento (Kraft)	1 oz.	117	.8

*Prepared as package directs.

Food and Description	Measure or Quantity	Calories	Carbohydrates (grams)
Tuna Salad (Carnation)	1/5 can	84	3.9
Turkey Salad (Carnation)	1/5 can	92	4.0
SAUCES & SAUCE MIXES			
Sauces, A1	1 tbsp.	14	3.4
Barbecue, Barbecue sauce (USDA)	1 cup	230	20
Hawaiian (Chun King)	1 tbsp.	16	3.5
Oven (Contadina)	1 fl. oz.	29	7.1
(French's)	1 tbsp.	9	2.1
Mild (French's)	1 tbsp.	17	4.1
Smoky (French's)	1 tbsp.	15	3.7
Hickory smoke, Open Pit (General Foods)	1 tbsp.	27	6.5
Hot 'n Spicy, Open Pit (General Foods)	1 tbsp.	27	6.3
Original flavor, Open Pit (General Foods)	1 tbsp.	26	6.3
Original flavor with onions, Open Pit (General Foods)	1 tbsp.	27	6.5
With onions, regular (Heinz)	1 tbsp.	19	4.2
With onions, hickory smoke (Heinz)	1 tbsp.	18	2.8
(Kraft)	1 oz.	34	7.9
Garlic (Kraft)	1 oz.	32	7.6
Hickory smoke (Kraft)	1 oz.	34	7.9
Hot (Kraft)	1 oz.	31	7.0
Mustard flavored (Kraft)	1 oz.	28	5.4
Onion (Kraft)	1 oz.	41	8.9
Brown, Canned (La Choy)	¼ cup	321	78.0
Cheese, Deluxe Dinner (Kraft)	1 oz.	77	2.0
Chili (USDA)	1 tbsp.	16	3.7
(Del Monte)	1 tbsp.	18	4.6
(Heinz)	1 tbsp.	17	3.8
(Hunt's)	1 tbsp.	19	4.9
(Stokely-Van Camp)	1 tbsp.	15	3.5
Chili Barbecue (Gebhardt)	1 oz.	14	3.0
Chutney (Spice Islands)	1 tbsp.	35	

193

Food and Description	Measure or Quantity	Calories	Carbohydrates (grams)
Creole (Contadina)	1 fl. oz.	14	2.4
Enchilada (Rosarita)	1 oz.	8	1.2
Escoffier Sauce Diable.	1 tbsp.	16	4.1
Escoffier Sauce Robert.	1 tbsp.	23	5.7
Famous (Durkee)	1 tbsp.	66	2.1
57 (Heinz)	1 tbsp.	14	2.6
Hard (Crosse & Blackwell)	1 tbsp.	64	8.3
Hollandaise (Cresca)	1 oz.	39	
Horseradish (Marzetti)	1 tbsp.	58	2.3
Hot (Gebhardt)	¼ tsp.	1	
H. P. Steak Sauce (Lea & Perrins)	1 tbsp.	20	4.8
Marinara (Buitoni)	4 oz.	67	8.0
(Chef-Boy-Ar-Dee)	¼ of 15-oz. can	68	10.9
Meat (Spice Islands)	1 tbsp.	25	
Meat loaf (Contadina)	1 fl. oz.	16	3.4
Mint (Crosse & Blackwell)	1 tbsp.	16	4.0
Mushroom (Contadina)	1 fl. oz.	22	2.4
Mustard (Spice Islands)	1 tbsp.	40	
Newburg, Canned (Snow)	4 oz.	129	8.7
Savory (Heinz)	1 tbsp.	20	4.5
Seafood cocktail			
(Crosse & Blackwell)	1 tbsp.	22	4.9
(Del Monte)	1 tbsp.	20	5.2
Shed's Old Style	1 tbsp.	48	1.5
Sloppy Joe (Contadina)	1 fl. oz.	18	4.0
Chili (Contadina)	1 fl. oz.	11	2.5
Pizza (Contadina)	1 fl. oz.	16	3.2
Soy (USDA)	1 oz.	19	2.7
All purpose (Chun King)	1 tbsp.	6	.3
Japanese style (Chun King)	1 tbsp.	5	.3
(La Choy)	¼ cup	51	4.0
Spaghetti Sauce, Clam, red			
(Buitoni)	4 oz.	106	1.4
Clam, white (Buitoni)	4 oz.	140	2.2
Italian (Contadina)	4 fl. oz.	76	12.0
Meat (Buitoni)	4 oz.	111	5.0
Meat (Chef-Boy-Ar-Dee)	¼ of 15-oz. can	93	10.1

Food and Description	Measure or Quantity	Cal- ories	Carbo- hydrates (grams)
Meat *(Heinz)*	½ cup	110	15.4
Meat *(Prince)*	½ cup	144	11.0
Meatball *(Chef-Boy-Ar-Dee)*	1/3 of 15-oz. can	202	21.2
With ground meat *(Chef-Boy-Ar-Dee)*	1/7 of 29-oz. jar	136	10.2
Meatless or plain *(Buitoni)*	4 oz.	76	9.5
Meatless or plain *(Chef-Boy-Ar-Dee)*	¼ of 16-oz. jar	73	12.4
Meatless or plain *(Heinz)*	½ cup	98	15.4
Meatless or plain *(Prince)*	½ cup	88	13.0
Meatless or plain *(Ronzoni)*	4 oz.	110	
Mushroom *(Buitoni)*	4 oz.	69	7.6
Mushroom *(Chef-Boy-Ar-Dee)*	¼ of 15-oz. can	68	11.4
Mushroom *(Heinz)*	½ cup	97	13.8
Mushroom with meat *(Heinz)*	½ cup	106	14.0
Steak *(Crosse & Blackwell)*	1 tbsp.	21	4.8
(Marzetti)	1 tbsp.	14	3.5
Stroganoff *(Contadina)*	1 fl. oz.	17	2.3
Sweet & Sour *(Chun King)*	1 tbsp.	52	12.6
Sweet & Sour *(Contadina)*	1 fl. oz.	37	7.7
Sweet & Sour *(Kraft)*	1 oz.	55	13.0
(La Choy)	¼ cup	122	27.5
Swiss Steak *(Contadina)*	1 fl. oz.	11	2.1
Taco *(Gebhardt)*	1 oz.	6	1.0
Tomato, Canned *(Contadina)*	1 cup	80	16.8
Canned, Plain *(Del Monte)*	1 cup	60	12.7
Canned, With mushrooms *(Del Monte)*	1 cup	75	17.0
Canned, With onions *(Del Monte)*	1 cup	90	18.5
Canned, With tomato tidbits *(Del Monte)*	1 cup	90	21.8
Canned, Plain *(Hunt's)*	1 cup	78	18.7
Canned, Herb *(Hunt's)*	1 cup	186	27.0

Food and Description	Measure or Quantity	Calories	Carbo- hydrates (grams)
Canned, Special (Hunt's)	1 cup	94	27.2
Canned, With bits (Hunt's)	1 cup	82	19.4
Canned, With cheese (Hunt's)	1 cup	107	20.6
Canned, With mushrooms (Hunt's)	1 cup	83	19.8
Tomato sauce with mushrooms (Hunt-Wesson)	4 oz.	40	9
Canned, With onions (Hunt's)	1 cup	102	24.5
Tomato Paste, Canned (USDA)	1 tbsp.	13	3.0
(Contadina)	6 oz.	150	35
Canned (Contadina)	1 tbsp.	24	4.9
(Del Monte)	6 oz.	150	34
Canned (Del Monte)	1 tbsp.	14	3.3
(Hunt-Wesson)	3 oz.	70	14
Canned (Hunt's)	1 tbsp.	14	3.2
Canned (Stokely-Van Camp)	1 tbsp.	106	24.1
Tomato Puree, Canned, regular pack (USDA)	1 cup	98	22.2
Canned, regular pack (Contadina)	1 cup	96	20.0
Canned, regular pack (Hunt's)	1 cup	92	21.9
Canned, dietetic pack (USDA)	8 oz.	88	20.0
Tartar, Regular (USDA)	1 tbsp.	74	.6
Low Calorie (USDA)	1 tbsp.	31	.9
(Bennett's)	1 tbsp.	80	.9
(Hellmann's /Best Foods)	1 tbsp.	70	0
(Kraft)	1 oz.	145	1.4
(Marzetti)	1 tbsp.	69	.8
(Mrs. Paul's)	4.2-oz. pkg.	668	8.0
Teriyaki (Chun King)	1 tbsp.	11	1.4
White, Thin, Home recipe (USDA)	1 cup	302	18.0
Medium, Home recipe (USDA)	1 cup	405	22
Thick, Home recipe (USDA)	1 cup	489	27.2
Worcestershire (Crosse & Blackwell)	1 tbsp.	15	3.6
(French's)	1 tbsp.	6	1.4
(Heinz)	1 tbsp.	11	2.5

Food and Description	Measure or Quantity	Calories	Carbohydrates (grams)
(Lea & Perrins)	1 tbsp.	12	3.0
À la King *(Durkee)	1 cup (1½-oz. pkg.)	273	25.5
Barbecue *(Kraft)	1 oz.	32	7.9
Bordelaise *(Betty Crocker)	¼ cup	33	5.2
Cheese *(Betty Crocker)	¼ cup	87	1.1
*(Durkee)	1 cup (1.4-oz. pkg.)	523	31.0
(French's)	1¼-oz. pkg.	165	11.2
Cheddar *(Kraft)	1 oz.	52	1.9
Hollandaise *(Betty Crocker)	¼ cup	84	4.0
*(Durkee)	2/3 cup	213	11.0
(French's)	1-1/8-oz. pkg.	192	6.8
*(Kraft)	1 oz.	54	2.0
*(McCormick)	2-oz. serving	73	4.0
Miracle (Mrs. Paul's)	½-oz. pkg.	10	2.1
Mushroom *(Betty Crocker)	¼ cup	36	5.0
Noodle-Roni *(Golden Grain)	½ cup	140	20.0
Newbury *(Betty Crocker)	¼ cup	68	5.9
Sloppy Joe, Mix, including seasoning mix (Durkee)	1½-oz. pkg.	76	18.7
Including seasoning mix, with tomato paste & meat *(Durkee)	3 cups	1432	50.3
Including seasoning mix (French's)	1½-oz. pkg.	117	26.0
Including seasoning mix *(Kraft)	1 oz.	47	1.8

* Prepared as package directs.

S
V

197

Food and Description	Measure or Quantity	Calories	Carbohydrates (grams)
Including seasoning mix (Lawry's)	1½-oz. pkg.	139	27.7
Including seasoning mix (McCormick)	1-5/16 oz. pkg.	112	
Including seasoning mix *(Wyler's)	6 fl. oz.	25	4.3
Sour Cream *(Durkee)	2/3 cup	325	30.0
(French's)	1¼-oz. pkg.	192	12.7
*(Kraft)	1 oz.	61	4.1
*(McCormick)	2-oz. serving	40	2.5
Stroganoff (French's)	1-¾-oz. pkg.	192	21.0
*(French's)	1/3 cup	104	9.3
Sweet-sour *(Durkee)	1 cup (2-oz. pkg.)	230	44.6
Tartar (Lawry's)	.6-oz. pkg.	64	9.8
Teriyaki *(Durkee)	3 cup (1¼-oz. pkg.)	66	15.9
White *(Durkee)	1 cup (1½-oz. pkg.)	381	25.0
*(Kraft)	1 oz.	44	2.5
Supreme *(McCormick)	2-oz. serving	22	4.0

SOUPS

Food and Description	Measure or Quantity	Calories	Carbohydrates (grams)
Alphabet, Soup mix *(Goodman's)	8 oz.	43	0
Asparagus Soup, Cream of, canned, condensed (USDA)	8 oz. by wt.	123	19.1
Canned, prepared with equal volume of water (USDA)	1 cup (8.5 oz.)	65	10.1

*Prepared as package directs.

Food and Description	Measure or Quantity	Calories	Carbohydrates (grams)
Canned, condensed, Cream of, prepared with equal volume of milk (USDA)	1 cup (8.5 oz.)	144	16.3
Canned, condensed, Cream of *(Campbell)	1 cup (8 oz.)	80	10.7
Bean Soup, Canned *(Manischewitz)	1 cup	111	17.6
Canned, with bacon *(Campbell)	1 cup	152	19.4
Canned, with smoked ham, "Great American" (Heinz)	1 cup (8-¾ oz.)	201	24.5
Bean Soup, Black, canned (Crosse & Blackwell)	6½ oz. ½ can	96	15.5
*(Campbell)	1 cup	91	13.9
Bean Soup, Lima, Canned *(Manischewitz)	1 cup	93	15.3
Bean with pork, canned (USDA)	1 cup	170	22
Beef Broth, bouillon, consomme, made with equal volume of water (USDA)	1 cup	30	3
Buillon, Canned (Campbell)	10 oz.	35	3
Beef Bouillon, Broth, Consomme, cubes or powder, instant (Croyden House)	1 tsp. (5 grams)	12	2.2
Beef Bouillon, Broth or Consomme, cubes or powder (Herb-Ox)	1 cube (4 grams)	6	.5
Instant (Herb-Ox)	1 packet (4 grams)	8	.8
*(Knovi Swiss)	6 fl. oz.	13	
Cube or instant (Maggi)	1 cube or 1 tsp. (4 grams)	7 7	.5 .5

*Prepared as package directs.

S
V

Food and Description	Measure or Quantity	Calories	Carbohydrates (grams)
(Steero)	1 cube (4 grams)	6	.5
Cube or instant (Wyler's)	1 cube	7	.4
	1 tsp.	7	.4
Beef Soup, Canned, broth (College Inn)	1 cup	19	5.2
Canned, broth (Swanson)	1 cup	18	.2
Canned *(Campbell)	1 cup	99	10.5
Canned, ready to serve, Chunky beef (Campbell)	9½ oz.	210	21
Canned, Chunky (Campbell)	1 cup	185	18.5
Barley, canned *(Manischewitz)	1 cup	83	11.2
Cabbage, canned *(Manischewitz)	1 cup	62	9.0
Beef Noodle, Canned made with equal volume of water (USDA)	1 cup	70	7
Canned (Campbell)	10 oz.	90	10
Canned *(Heinz)	1 cup (8.5 oz.)	74	6.7
Canned *(Manischewitz)	1 cup	64	8.0
Sirloin burger, Chunky, canned (Campbell)	1 cup	162	14.3
Vegetable, canned *(Manischewitz)	1 cup	59	8.9
Beef Soup Mix, Barley *(Wyler's)	6 fl. oz.	54	9.3
Broth, Cup-a-Soup (Lipton)	1 pkg. (8 grams)	19	3.6
Noodle (USDA)	1 oz.	110	18.5
Noodle, Cup-a-Soup (Lipton)	1 pkg. (4 oz.)	34	6.3
Noodle, with vegetable *(Lipton)	1 cup	66	11.0
Noodle *(Wyler's)	6 fl. oz.	37	7.0
Beef with Dumplings, "Great American" (Heinz)	1 cup (8-¾ oz.)	109	11.1

*Prepared as package directs.

Food and Description	Measure or Quantity	Calories	Carbohydrates (grams)
Borscht (Manischewitz)	1 cup	72	17.5
(Manischewitz)	1 cup	48	
Regular (Mother's)	1 cup	40	
Bouillon, Bouillon cubes, approx. ½ in. (USDA)	1 cube	5	Trace
Celery Soup, Cream of, Condensed, made with equal volume of milk (Campbell)	1 cup	75	7.3
(Heinz)	1 cup	101	9.0
Clam Chowder, Manhattan type, With tomatoes, without milk, canned, made with equal volume of water (USDA)	1 cup	80	12
Manhattan style, canned, made with equal volume of water (Campbell)	10 oz.	100	15
Canned, made with equal volume of water (Doxsee)	8 oz.	100	18
New England, canned, made with equal volume of water (Campbell)	10 oz.	100	13
New England, with milk, canned (Doxsee)	8 oz.	190	27
Chicken, & Noodle, canned, condensed (USDA)	8 oz.	120	15.0
Barley, canned *(Manischewitz)	1 cup	83	12.3
Gumbo, canned *(Campbell)	1 cup	55	8.3
With rice, canned *(Campbell)	1 cup	49	5.6
With stars, canned *(Heinz)	1 cup	66	7.9
Chunky Chicken, canned (Campbell)	9½ oz.	200	20
Cream of chicken, canned, made with equal volume of water (USDA)	1 cup	95	8

* Prepared as package directs.

S V

Food and Description	Measure or Quantity	Cal- ories	Carbo- hydrates (grams)
Canned, made with equal volume of water *(Campbell)*	10 oz.	140	10
Canned, condensed, with equal volume of milk *(USDA)*	1 cup	180	15
Chili Beef, canned *(Campbell)*	1 cup	149	20.8
(Heinz)	1 cup	161	21.2
"Great American" *(Heinz)*	1 cup	179	22.0
Crab *(Crosse & Blackwell)*	½ can	59	8.3
Dehydrated, Chicken noodle with meat *(Lipton)*	1 cup	70	9
Chicken rice *(Lipton)*	1 cup	60	8
Noodle soup *(Lipton)*	1 cup	50	7
Onion soup *(Lipton)*	1 cup	35	6
Tomato vegetable *(Lipton)*	1 cup	70	12
Vegetable beef *(Lipton)*	1 cup	60	8
Lobster, Cream of, canned *(Crosse & Blackwell)*	½ can	92	6.5
Minestrone, canned, made with equal volume of water *(Campbell)*	10 oz.	110	15
Canned, made with equal volume of water *(USDA)*	1 cup	105	14
Mushroom, Cream of, canned, condensed, with equal volume of milk *(USDA)*	1 cup	215	16
Cream of, canned, made with equal volume of water *(Campbell)*	10 oz.	150	11
Cream of, canned, made with equal volume of water *(USDA)*	1 cup	135	10
Oyster Stew, Home recipe, 1 part oysters to 1 part milk by volume *(USDA)*	1 cup	245	14.2
Home recipe, 1 part oysters to 3 parts milk by volume *(USDA)*	1 cup	233	10.8

*Prepared as package directs.

Food and Description	Measure or Quantity	Calories	Carbohydrates (grams)
Home recipe, 1 part oysters to 3 parts milk by volume (USDA)	1 cup	206	11.3
Canned *(Campbell)	1 cup	142	11.6
Frozen, condensed, made with equal volume of water (USDA)	1 cup	122	8.2
Frozen, condensed, made with equal volume of milk (USDA)	1 cup	202	14.2
Shrimp, Cream of, canned *(Campbell)	1 cup	171	12.8
Cream of, canned (Crosse & Blackwell)	½ can	92	6.5
Frozen, condensed (USDA)	8 oz.	302	16.3
Frozen, condensed, made with equal volume of water (USDA)	1 cup	158	8.4
Frozen, condensed, made with equal volume of milk (USDA)	1 cup	243	15.2
Split pea, canned, made with equal volume of water (USDA)	1 cup	145	21
Split pea with ham, canned, made with equal volume of water (Campbell)	10 oz.	210	30
Tomato, Canned, made with equal volume of water (USDA)	1 cup	90	16
Canned, condensed, regular pack, made with equal volume of water (USDA)	1 cup	88	15.7
Cream of, canned, condensed, made with equal volume of milk (USDA)	1 cup	175	23
Canned, made with equal volume of water (Campbell)	10 oz.	110	20

*Prepared as package directs.

203

S
V

Food and Description	Measure or Quantity	Calories	Carbo-hydrates (grams)
Canned, condensed, regular pack, California *(Heinz)	1 cup	79	14.0
Canned, "Great American" (Heinz)	1 cup	87	18.3
Canned, condensed *(Manischewitz)	1 cup	60	9.1
Beef, Noodle-O's *(Campbell)	1 cup	109	15.5
Bisque *(Campbell)	1 cup	115	20.9
Rice, old-fashioned *(Campbell)	1 cup	99	16.7
Tomato made with milk, Canned, condensed (Campbell)	10 oz.	210	27
Tomato Rice *(Manischewitz)	1 cup	78	12.8
Tomato with vegetables, "Great American" (Heinz)	1 cup	126	17.6
Tomato, Dietetic pack, low sodium, canned (Campbell)	7¼-oz. can	97	16.9
Dietetic pack, with rice, canned *(Claybourne)	8 oz.	73	14.6
Dietetic pack, with rice, canned *(Slim-ette)	8 oz.	34	7.2
Dietetic pack, canned (Tillie Lewis)	1 cup	70	11.8
Vegetable, Chunky vegetable, canned, ready to serve (Campbell)	9½ oz.	140	22
Vegetarian vegetable, canned, made with equal volume of water (Campbell)	10 oz.	90	16
Vegetarian, canned, made with equal volume of water (USDA)	1 cup	80	13
Vegetable beef, canned, made with equal volume of water (USDA)	1 cup	80	10
Vegetable beef, canned, made with equal volume of water (Campbell)	10 oz.	90	10

*Prepared as package directs.

Food and Description	Measure or Quantity	Calories	Carbohydrates (grams)
SOUP MIX			
Chicken, Broth, Cup-a-Broth			
(Lipton)	1 pkg.	23	3.2
Consomme *(Knorr Swiss)*	6 fl. oz.	11	
Cream of, Cup-a-Broth			
(Lipton)	1 pkg.	95	9.7
Chicken & Noodle *(USDA)*	2-oz. pkg.	218	33.1
(Golden Grain)	1 cup	58	8.8
(Lipton)	1 cup	53	7.2
(Wyler's)	6 fl. oz.	33	4.2
Cup-a-Soup *(Lipton)*	1 pkg.	37	5.9
Giggle *(Lipton)*	1 cup	76	11.3
Ring-O-Noodle *(Lipton)*	1 cup	57	9.4
With diced chicken *(Lipton)*	1 cup	68	8.9
With meat, Cup-a-Soup			
(Lipton)	.4-oz. pkg.	42	5.8
Chicken & Rice *(USDA)*	1 cup	46	8.0
(Lipton)	1 cup	63	7.9
Rice-A-Roni.	1 cup	63	10.9
(Wyler's)	6 fl. oz.	37	6.4
Tomato, Cup-a-Soup *(Lipton)*	1 pkg.	79	17.3
Vegetable with noodles *(USDA)*	1 oz.	98	17.8
Vegetable with noodles			
(Golden Grain)	1 cup	80	13.3
Vegetable with noodles			
(Lipton)	1 cup	68	11.7
SUGARS, SWEETS, SYRUPS, ICINGS			
Sugar, Brown *(USDA)*	1 lb.	1692	437.3
Brown, firm packed *(USDA)*	1 cup	820	121
	1 tbsp.	48	12.5
Brownulated *(USDA)*	1 cup	567	146.5
Confectioners *(USDA)*	1 lb.	1746	451.3
Confectioners, Unsifted *(USDA)*	1 cup	474	122.4
	1 tbsp.	30	7.7
Confectioners, Sifted *(USDA)*	1 cup	462	119.4
	1 tbsp.	29	7.5

*Prepared as package directs.

SV

Food and Description	Measure or Quantity	Calories	Carbohydrates (grams)
Granulated (USDA)	1 lump	23	6.0
Maple (USDA)	1 lb.	1579	408.0
Maple (USDA)	1 piece (1.2 oz.)	104	27.0
Powdered, Stirred before measuring (USDA)	1 cup	460	119
	1 tbsp.	29	7.5
White, granulated (USDA)	1 cup	770	199
	1 lb.	1746	451.3
White, granulated (USDA)	1 tbsp.	40	11
Sugar Substitute (Weight Watchers)	1 packet	4	.9
(Adolph's)	1 tsp.	0	0
Sweetnin' (Tillie Lewis)	1 tsp.	0	0
Sweets, Honey, strained or extracted (USDA)	½ cup	496	134.1
Honey, strained (USDA)	1 tbsp.	61	16.5
Molasses, blackstrap (USDA)	1 tbsp.	45	11
Molasses, cane, light (USDA)	1 tbsp.	50	13
Syrup, Chocolate-flavored syrup, fudge type (USDA)	1 fl. oz.	125	20
Chocolate-flavored syrup (Hershey)	1 oz. (2 tbsp.)	90	22
Chocolate-flavored syrup (Bosco)	1 tbsp.	50	13
Chocolate-flavored syrup or topping, thin type (USDA)	1 fl. oz.	90	24
Corn syrup, light (Karo)	1 tbsp.	60	15
	1 cup	949	237.2
Corn syrup, dark (Karo)	1 tbsp.	60	15
	1 cup	956	239.0
Imitation maple syrup (Karo)	1 tbsp.	60	15
	1 cup	933	233.0
Log Cabin, Buttered.	1 tbsp.	46	12.2
Log Cabin, Country Kitchen, pancake & waffle.	1 tbsp.	51	13.1
Log Cabin, Maple-honey.	1 tbsp.	54	14.0

Food and Description	Measure or Quantity	Calories	Carbo-hydrates (grams)
Log Cabin, Regular.	1 tbsp.	46	12.2
Pancake syrup (S & W Nutradiet)	1 tsp.	4	1
Pancake syrup (Golden Griddle)	1 tbsp.	50	13
Pancake & Waffle syrup (Karo)	1 tbsp.	60	15
	1 cup	949	236.9
Sorghum (USDA)	1 tbsp.	55	14
Syrup (Aunt Jemima)	¼ cup	212	54
Table blend (USDA)	1 tbsp.	60	14
Cake Icing, Butterscotch (Betty Crocker)	1/12 of 16.5-oz. can	164	27.8
Caramel, Home recipe (USDA)	4 oz.	408	86.8
Cherry (Betty Crocker)	1/12 of 16.5-oz. can	167	28.0
Chocolate, Home recipe (USDA)	1 cup	1034	185.4
Chocolate icing made with milk & table fat (USDA)	1 cup	1035	185
Chocolate fudge, ready to spread (Pillsbury)	1/12 can	160	24
Chocolate, ready to spread (Betty Crocker)	1/12 can	170	25
Coconut, with boiled icing (USDA)	1 cup	605	124
Lemon, ready to spread (Pillsbury)	(for 1/12 cake) 1/12 of 16.5--oz. can	160	27
Milk Chocolate (Betty Crocker)	1/12 can	164	27.2
Orange, ready to spread (Betty Crocker)	1/12 can	160	26
Vanilla (Betty Crocker)	1/12 can	166	28.0
White, boiled icing, home recipe (USDA)	1 cup	300	76

S V

Food and Description	Measure or Quantity	Calories	Carbohydrates (grams)
White, uncooked, home recipe *(USDA)*	4 oz.	426	92.5
Cake Icing Mix, Banana *(Betty Crocker)*	1/12 of icing	139	29.5
Butter Brickle *(Betty Crocker)*	1/12 of icing	140	29.7
Caramel *(Betty Crocker)*	1/12 of icing	139	29.6
Caramel apple *(Betty Crocker)*	12 of icing	130	29.5
Cherry, creamy *(Betty Crocker)*	1/12 of icing	139	29.3
Cherry fluff *(Betty Crocker)*	1/12 of icing	59	16.6
Cherry Fudge *(Betty Crocker)*	1/12 of icing	132	28.5
Chocolate fudge *(Pillsbury)*	for 1/12 cake	170	28
Chocolate fudge, creamy *(Betty Crocker)*	1/12 pkg.	160	32
Chocolate malt *(Betty Crocker)*	1/12 of icing	136	28.7
Chocolate walnut *(Betty Crocker)*	1/12 of icing	131	26.6
Coconut-pecan *(Betty Crocker)*	1/12 of icing	102	16.6
Coconut, toasted *(Betty Crocker)*	1/12 of icing	141	28.7
Creamy Fudge, from mix with water only *(USDA)*	1 cup	830	183

*Prepared as package directs.

Food and Description	Measure or Quantity	Calories	Carbo-hydrates (grams)
Dark chocolate fudge *(Betty Crocker)	1/12 of icing	130	27.4
Fluffy chocolate *(Betty Crocker)	1/12 pkg.	80	13
Fluffy white (Pillsbury)	for 1/12 cake	70	17
Fluffy white *(Betty Crocker)	1/12 pkg.	60	16
Fudge, creamy, contains nonfat dry milk, prepared with water & fat (USDA)	8 oz.	869	149.5
Lemon (Pillsbury)	for 1/12 cake	160	29
Lemon fluff *(Betty Crocker)	1/12 of icing	58	14.9
Milk chocolate *(Betty Crocker)	1/12 of icing	130	28.9
Orange *(Betty Crocker)	1/12 of icing	134	28.9
Orange, creamy *(Betty Crocker)	1/12 pkg.	150	30
Pineapple *(Betty Crocker)	1/12 of icing	134	28.4
Sour cream, chocolate fudge *(Betty Crocker)	1/12 of icing	129	27.5
Sour cream, white *(Betty Crocker)	1/12 of icing	130	29.0
Spice, creamy *(Betty Crocker)	1/12 of icing	139	29.2
White, creamy *(Betty Crocker)	1/12 pkg.	160	33

* Prepared as package directs.

S
V

Food and Description	Measure or Quantity	Calories	Carbohydrates (grams)
VEGETABLES			
Artichoke, Globe or French, hearts, frozen *(Bird's Eye)*	5-6 hearts or 3 oz.	22	4.8
Globe or French, boiled, drained *(USDA)*	4 oz.	50	11.2
Globe or French, whole, raw *(USDA)*	1 lb. weighed untrimmed	85	19.2
Jerusalem Artichoke, pared *(USDA)*	4 oz.	75	18.9
Jerusalem Artichoke, unpared *(USDA)*	1 lb. weighed with skin	207	52.3
Asparagus, Canned, solids and liquid *(USDA)*	1 cup	45	7
All green *(S & W Nutradiet)*	½ cup	17	3
Green, cooked, drained, pieces 1½ to 2 in. lengths *(USDA)*	1 cup	30	5
Green, cooked, drained, spears ½ in. diam. at base *(USDA)*	4 spears	10	2
Cut spears *(Green Giant)*	1 cup	40	5
Spears *(Le Sueur)*	1 cup	40	5
Cut spears in butter, frozen, Boil-in-Bag *(Green Giant)*	1 cup	90	7
Spears, frozen *(Bird's Eye)*	3.3 oz.	25	3
Spears with Hollandaise sauce *(Bird's Eye)*	1/3 pkg. (3.3 oz.)	97	3.2
White, spears & liquid *(USDA)*	4 oz.	20	3.7
White, spears only *(USDA)*	6 med. spears	21	3.5
White, spears only *(Del Monte)*	1 cup (7.6 oz.)	39	7.3
Bamboo Shoot, Canned, sliced *(La Choy)*	1 cup	12	2.0

Food and Description	Measure or Quantity	Calories	Carbohydrates (grams)
Raw, untrimmed *(USDA)*	½ lb. (weighed untrimmed)	18	3.4
Raw, trimmed *(USDA)*	4 oz.	31	5.9
Bavarian-Style Beans & Spaetzle, Frozen *(Bird's Eye)*	1/3 pkg. (3-1/3 oz.)	135	11.8
Beans, Baked, Canned in molasses sauce & brown sugar sauce *(Campbell)*	1 cup	310	48.1
Canned with brown sugar sauce, Yellow eye bean *(B & M)*	1 cup (8 oz.)	359	50.6
Canned in molasses sauce *(Heinz)*	1 cup (9¼ oz.)	283	52.8
Canned with pork, Home Style *(Campbell)*	1 cup	302	52.0
Canned with pork, Snack Pack *(Hunt's)*	5-oz. can	169	35.3
Canned with pork *(Van Camp)*	1 cup (7.7 oz.)	286	41.8
Canned with pork & molasses sauce *(USDA)*	1 cup (9 oz.)	382	53.8
Canned with pork & molasses sauce, Michigan Pea, New England-style *(B & M)*	1 cup (7.9 oz.)	336	50.8
Canned with pork & molasses sauce, Michigan Pea, New England-style *(Homemaker's)*	1 cup (8 oz.)	320	48.8
Canned with pork & molasses sauce, Boston-style *(Heinz)*	1 cup (8¾ oz.)	303	50.8
Canned with pork & tomato sauce *(USDA)*	1 cup (9 oz.)	311	48.4

Food and Description	Measure or Quantity	Calories	Carbohydrates (grams)
Canned with pork & tomato sauce (Campbell)	1 cup	262	42.7
Canned with pork & tomato sauce (Heinz)	1 cup (9¼ oz.)	293	48.5
Canned with pork & tomato sauce (Libby's)	1 cup (9.3 oz.)	286	52.7
Canned with tomato sauce (USDA)	1 cup (9 oz.)	306	58.6
Canned with tomato sauce, Campside (Heinz)	1 cup (9½ oz.)	350	51.1
Canned with tomato sauce, Vegetarian (Heinz)	1 cup (9¼ oz.)	267	48.9
Canned with tomato sauce (Van Camp)	1 cup (8.1 oz.)	276	52.0
Bean, Barbecue (Campbell)	1 cup	287	51.1
Bean, Black, Dry (USDA)	4 oz.	384	69.4
Bean, Brown, Dry (USDA)	4 oz.	384	69.4
Bean, Calico, Dry (USDA)	4 oz.	396	72.2
Beans, Dry, Common varieties, cooked, drained, Great Northern (USDA)	1 cup	210	38
Cooked, drained, Great Northern (Kounty Kist)	1 cup	180	32
Cooked, drained, Navy (pea) (USDA)	1 cup	225	40
Cooked, drained, Pea Beans (B & M Baked Beans)	1 oz.	42	6.4
Cooked, drained, White or Pea Beans (Kounty Kist)	1 cup	190	34
Beans, Canned, Solids & Liquid, Barbecue beans (Campbell)	8 oz.	280	46
Chili beans (Hunt's)	1 cup	234	41.7

Food and Description	Measure or Quantity	Calories	Carbohydrates (grams)
Home-style beans *(Campbell)*	8 oz.	300	52
Kidney beans *(Hunt's)*	1 cup	237	44.5
Dark red kidney beans *(Kounty Kist)*	1 cup	190	36
Light red kidney beans *(Kounty Kist)*	1 cup	210	40
Red kidney beans *(USDA)*	1 cup	230	42
Red kidney beans *(B & M Baked Beans)*	1 oz.	45	6.2
Red kidney beans, canned with brown sugar sauce *(B & M)*	1 cup (8 oz.)	360	49.7
(Homemaker's)	1 cup (8 oz.)	337	50.2
Old fashioned beans in molasses and brown sugar sauce *(Campbell)*	8 oz.	290	49
Oven baked beans in tomato sauce *(Morton House)*	4 oz.	140	23
Pork & Beans with tomato sauce *(Campbell)*	8 oz.	260	44
Pork & Beans *(Hunt's)*	8 oz.	289	55.2
Pork & Beans *(Kounty Kist)*	1 cup	250	42
Small red beans *(Hunt's)*	1 cup	220	40.7
White beans with frankfurters, sliced *(USDA)*	1 cup	365	32
White beans with pork and sweet sauce *(USDA)*	1 cup	385	54
White beans with pork and tomato sauce *(USDA)*	1 cup	310	49
Bean & Frankfurter, Canned *(USDA)*	1 cup (9 oz.)	367	32.1
Canned, in molasses & sauce *(Campbell)*	1 cup	364	35.7
Canned *(Heinz)*	1 cup (8-¾ oz.)	399	38.0

213

Food and Description	Measure or Quantity	Calories	Carbohydrates (grams)
Canned, Beanie-Weenee (Van Camp)	1 cup (7.8 oz.)	316	27.6
Bean, Green or Snap, Fresh, whole (USDA)	1 lb. (weighed untrimmed)	128	28.3
1½ to 2 in. pieces, fresh, whole (USDA)	½ cup (1.8 oz.)	17	3.7
French-style, fresh, whole (USDA)	½ cup (1.4 oz.)	13	2.8
Boiled, drained, fresh, whole (USDA)	½ cup (2.2 oz.)	16	3.3
1½ to 2 in. pieces, drained, fresh, boiled (USDA)	½ cup (2.4 oz.)	17	3.7
Canned, regular pack, cut, solids & liquid (Comstock-Greenwood)	½ cup (3 oz.)	20	4.4
Canned, regular pack, solids & liquid (Stokely-Van Camp)	½ cup (3.9 oz.)	20	4.6
Canned, regular pack, drained solids (Butter Kernel)	½ cup (3.9 oz.)	20	4.6
Canned, seasoned, solids & liquid (Del Monte)	½ cup (4 oz.)	19	4.3
Canned, seasoned, drained solids (Del Monte)	½ cup (2.5 oz.)	15	2.6
Canned, with bacon (Comstock-Greenwood)	4 oz.	26	7.7

Food and Description	Measure or Quantity	Calories	Carbohydrates (grams)
Canned, with mushroom, solids & liquid (Comstock-Greenwood)	4 oz.	15	2.9
Canned, dietetic pack, solids & liquid (USDA)	4 oz.	18	4.1
Canned, dietetic pack, drained solids (USDA)	4 oz.	25	5.4
Canned, dietetic pack, drained liquid (USDA)	4 oz.	9	2.0
Canned, dietetic pack, cut, solids & liquid (Blue Boy)	4 oz.	26	5.3
Canned, dietetic pack, solids & liquid (Diet Delight)	½ cup (4.2 oz.)	20	3.6
Canned, dietetic pack, solids & liquid (Tillie Lewis)	½ cup (4.2 oz.)	20	3.6
Frozen, whole (Bird's Eye)	1/3 pkg. (3 oz.)	23	5.2
Frozen, cut, not thawed (USDA)	10-oz. pkg.	74	17.0
Frozen, cut, boiled, drained (USDA)	4 oz.	28	6.5
Frozen, cut (Bird's Eye)	1/3 pkg. (3 oz.)	22	5.1
Frozen, French-style, boiled, drained (USDA)	½ cup (2.8 oz.)	21	4.8
Frozen, French-style with sliced mushrooms (Bird's Eye)	1/3 pkg. (3 oz.)	26	5.5
Frozen, French-style with toasted almonds (Bird's Eye)	½ cup (3 oz.)	52	6.0
Green beans, Cut French-style in butter sauce, frozen, Boil-in-Bag (Green Giant)	1 cup	70	7
Mushroom sauce, onions, casserole (Green Giant)	1 cup	100	14

Food and Description	Measure or Quantity	Calories	Carbohydrates (grams)
Onions, bacon bits in light sauce, frozen, Boil-in-Bag (*Green Giant*)	1 cup	70	8
Cut, in mushroom sauce, frozen, Boil-in-Bag (*Green Giant*)	1 cup	90	14
Italian beans (*Del Monte*)	1 cup	60	11
Italian green beans, Frozen (*Bird's Eye*)	3 oz.	30	6
In tomato sauce, frozen, Boil-in-Bag (*Green Giant*)	1 cup	110	16
Bean, Kidney or Red, Canned, solids & liquid (*USDA*)	½ cup (4.5 oz.)	115	21.0
Canned, drained solids (*Butter Kernel*)	½ cup (4.2 oz.)	108	19.7
Canned, Red Kidney & Chili gravy (*Nalley's*)	4 oz.	120	18.5
Bean, Lima, Immature seeds, cooked, drained (*USDA*)	1 cup	190	34
Young, raw, whole (*USDA*)	1 lb. (weighed in pod)	223	40.1
Young, raw, without shell (*USDA*)	1 lb. (weighed shelled)	558	100.2
Young, raw, boiled, drained (*USDA*)	½ cup (3 oz.)	94	16.8
Cooked, drained (*USDA*)	1 cup	260	49
Canned, regular pack, solids & liquid (*USDA*)	½ cup (4.4 oz.)	88	16.6
Canned, regular pack, seasoned, drained solids (*Del Monte*)	½ cup (3.1 oz.)	88	15.8

Food and Description	Measure or Quantity	Calories	Carbohydrates (grams)
Canned, dietetic pack, drained solids, low sodium *(USDA)*	4 oz.	108	20.1
Solids & liquid *(Libby's)*	1 cup	160	30
(Del Monte)	1 cup	150	29
Canned, dietetic pack, solids & liquid, unseasoned *(Blue Bay)*	4 oz.	79	12.6
Frozen *(Fordhook)*	3.3 oz.	100	18
Bean, Baby Lima, Frozen *(Bird's Eye)*	3.3 oz.	120	22
Frozen, Poly Bag *(Green Giant)*	1 cup	150	28
In butter sauce, frozen, Boil-in-Bag *(Green Giant)*	1 cup	220	32
Bean, Baby Butter, Frozen *(Bird's Eye)*	3.3 oz.	130	24
Bean, Pinto, Dry *(USDA)*	4 oz.	396	72.2
Bean Salad, 3 Bean salad *(Green Giant)*	1 cup	220	45
Canned, solids & liquid *(Comstock-Greenwood)*	4 oz.	81	7.5
Canned, solids & liquid, Snack Pack *(Hunt's)*	5-oz. can	111	23.7
Canned, solids & liquid *(Le Sueur)*	¼ of 1 lb. 1-oz. can	75	15.1
Bean, Snap, Green beans, Whole, frozen *(Bird's Eye)*	3 oz.	25	5
Green beans, cut *(S & W Nutradiet)*	½ cup	20	4
Green beans, cooked, drained *(USDA)*	1 cup	30	7
Green beans, canned, solids & liquid *(USDA)*	1 cup	45	10
Green beans, cut *(Del Monte)*	1 cup	40	8
Green beans, whole, cut French-style *(Green Giant)*	1 cup	30	6
Green beans, Blue Lake, cut or whole, solids & liquid *(Libby's)*	1 cup	40	8

Food and Description	Measure or Quantity	Cal-ories	Carbo-hydrates (grams)
Green beans, Blue Lake, French-style, solids & liquid (Libby's)	1 cup	35	8
Green beans, whole (Del Monte)	1 cup	35	6
Bean Sprout, Mung, raw (USDA)	½ lb.	80	15.0
Sprouted mung beans, cooked, drained (USDA)	1 cup	35	7
Soy, raw (USDA)	½ lb.	104	12.0
Soy, boiled, drained (USDA)	4 oz.	43	4.2
Wax Beans, Whole, cut French-style (Green Giant)	1 cup	30	6
Solids & liquid (Libby's)	1 cup	40	9
Frozen, cut (Bird's Eye)	3 oz.	30	4
Yellow or Wax Beans, Raw, whole (USDA)	1 lb. (weighed untrimmed)	108	24.0
Wax beans, cooked, drained (USDA)	1 cup	30	6
Wax beans, canned, solids & liquid (USDA)	1 cup	45	10
Wax beans, cut (Del Monte)	1 cup	35	7
Canned, dietetic pack, solids & liquid (USDA)	4oz.	17	3.9
Beets, Cooked, drained, peeled, whole, 2 in. diam. (USDA)	2 beets	30	7
Diced or sliced (USDA)	1 cup	55	12
Canned, solids & liquid.	1 cup	85	19
Cut, sliced or whole (Del Monte)	1 cup	70	15
Sliced or cut, whole, solids & liquid brine pack (Libby's)	1 cup	70	16
Sliced (S & W Nutradiet)	½ cup	35	9
Whole, rosebud (Aunt Nellie's)	1 cup	80	18
Pickled, crinkle cut (Del Monte)	1 cup	150	36
Pickled, solids & liquid (Libby's)	1 cup	150	37

Food and Description	Measure or Quantity	Calories	Carbo-hydrates (grams)
Tiny, whole, solids & liquid _(Le Sueur)_	¼ of 1-lb. can	37	9.1
Harvard, solids & liquid _(Libby's)_	1 cup	160	40
Shoestring, solids & liquid _(Libby's)_	1 cup	50	12
Sweet sour, Harvard _(Aunt Nellie's)_	1 cup	210	51
Dietetic pack, sliced, unseasoned _(S & W Nutradiet)_	4 oz.	32	7.3
Dietetic pack, diced, solids & liquid _(Tillie Lewis)_	½ cup (4.3 oz.)	40	9.0
Frozen, sliced in orange flavor glaze _(Bird's Eye)_	1/3 of pkg. (3.3 oz.)	54	14.9
Beet greens, Leaves & stems, cooked, drained _(USDA)_	1 cup	25	5
Broccoli, Chopped, yield from 10-oz. frozen pkg. _(USDA)_	1-3/8 cup	65	12
Chopped, frozen _(Bird's Eye)_	3.3 oz.	25	4
Cooked, drained, whole stalks, medium size _(USDA)_	1 stalk	45	8
Cooked, drained, stalks cut into ½ in. pieces _(USDA)_	1 cup	40	7
Cut, Poly Bag _(Green Giant)_	1 cup	30	5
Cut spears in cheese sauce, frozen _(Green Giant)_	1 cup	130	13
Spears, frozen _(Bird's Eye)_	3.3 oz.	25	4
Spears in butter sauce, frozen _(Green Giant)_	1 cup	90	8
Broccoli Amandine, Frozen casserole _(Green Giant)_	1 cup	140	16
Brussel Sprouts, 7 to 8 sprouts, (1¼ to 1½ in. diam.) cooked.	1 cup	55	10
Au gratin, casserole _(Green Giant)_	1 cup	160	17
Frozen _(Bird's Eye)_	3.3 oz.	25	4

S
V

219

Food and Description	Measure or Quantity	Calories	Carbohydrates (grams)
Frozen, Poly Bag (Green Giant)	1 cup	50	8
In butter sauce, frozen (Green Giant)	1 cup	110	10
Cabbage, Finely shredded or chopped, cooked (USDA)	1 cup	30	6
Finely shredded, or chopped, raw (USDA)	1 cup	20	5
Coarsely shredded or sliced, raw (USDA)	1 cup	15	4
Spoon (or Pak-Choy) cooked (USDA)	1 cup	25	4
Cabbage, Red, Canned (Comstock-Greenwood)	4 oz.	77	18.0
Raw, coarsely shredded (USDA)	1 cup (2.5 oz.)	22	4.8
Cabbage, Savoy, Raw, coarsely shredded (USDA)	1 cup (2.5 oz.)	17	3.2
California Blend, Broccoli, cauliflower, carrots, frozen (Green Giant)	1 cup	30	5
Carrots, Canned, diced or sliced (Del Monte)	1 cup	60	15
Canned, diced or sliced (Libby's)	1 cup	40	9
Cooked, diced (USDA)	1 cup	45	10
Crinkle cut, honey glazed, frozen (Green Giant)	1 cup	170	30
Nuggets in butter sauce, frozen (Green Giant)	1 cup	100	12
Raw, grated (USDA)	1 cup	45	11
Raw, whole, 5½ in. by 1 in. (25 thin strips) (USDA)	1 carrot	20	5
Sliced (S & W Nutradiet)	½ cup	30	7
Cauliflower, Cooked, flower buds (USDA)	1 cup	25	5
Frozen (Bird's Eye)	3.3 oz.	25	4
Frozen, Poly Bag (Green Giant)	1 cup	25	4

Food and Description	Measure or Quantity	Cal-ories	Carbo-hydrates (grams)
Hungarian Cauliflower, frozen casserole (Green Giant)	1 cup	130	14
In butter sauce, frozen (Green Giant)	1 cup	80	6
In cheese sauce, frozen (Green Giant)	1 cup	150	15
Celeriac Root, Raw, whole (USDA)	1 lb. (weighed unpared)	156	33.2
Raw, pared (USDA)	4 oz.	45	9.6
Celery, Boiled, drained (USDA)	½ cup	11	2.4
Raw pieces, diced (USDA)	1 cup	15	4
Raw, stalk, large outer, 8 in. by about 1½ in. at root end (USDA)	1 stalk	5	2
Celery, or Chinese Cabbage, Raw, cut in 1 in. pieces (USDA)	1 cup	10	2
Chicory Greens, Raw, untrimmed (USDA)	½ lb.	37	7.0
Chicory, Witloaf, Belgian or French endive, raw, bleached head, untrimmed (USDA)	½ lb.	30	6.4
Chives, Raw (USDA)	1 oz.	8	1.6
Collards, Cooked (USDA)	1 cup	55	9
Chopped, collard greens, frozen (Bird's Eye)	3.3 oz.	30	4
Corn, Canned, solids & liquid (USDA)	1 cup	170	40
Fritter, frozen (Mrs. Paul's)	2 fritters	260	31
'N' Peppers (Del Monte)	1 cup	190	40
On the cob, frozen (Bird's Eye)	1 ear	130	28
Cream style (S & W Nutradiet)	½ cup	100	21
Golden cream style (Del Monte)	1 cup	210	46
Golden cream style (Green Giant)	1 cup	210	45
Golden family style (Del Monte)	1 cup	170	37

Food and Description	Measure or Quantity	Calories	Carbohydrates (grams)
Golden vacuum packed (Del Monte)	1 cup	200	43
Golden, whole kernel, liquid pack (Green Giant)	1 cup	160	33
Golden, whole kernel, liquid pack (LeSueur)	1 cup	170	35
Golden, whole kernel, frozen (Green Giant)	1 cup	130	26
Golden, in butter sauce, frozen (Niblets)	1 cup	190	30
Golden corn on cob, frozen (Green Giant)	5½ in. ear	160	33
	3 in. coblet	90	18
Golden corn/peppers in butter sauce (Mexicorn)	1 cup	190	30
Scalloped corn casserole, frozen (Green Giant)	1 cup	330	40
Sweet, cooked, ear 5 in. by 1-¾ in. (USDA)	1 ear	70	16
Sweet, cream style (Libby's)	1 cup	170	42
Sweet whole kernel corn, frozen (Bird's Eye)	3.3 oz.	30	5
White, cream style (Del Monte)	1 cup	190	42
White whole kernel (Del Monte)	1 cup	150	33
White whole kernel, vacuum pack (Green Giant)	1 cup	150	30
White whole kernel, frozen (Green Giant)	1 cup	130	26
White whole kernel in butter sauce, frozen (Mexicorn)	1 cup	190	30
Whole kernel (S & W Nutradiet)	½ cup	80	15
Whole kernel, wet pack (Libby's)	1 cup	160	37
Cowpeas, Cooked, immature seeds (USDA)	1 cup	175	29
Cucumbers, 10 oz., 7½ in. by about 2 in., raw, pared (USDA)	1 cucumber	30	7
Dandelion greens, Cooked (USDA)	1 cup	60	12

Food and Description	Measure or Quantity	Cal- ories	Carbo- hydrates (grams)
Eggplant, Cooked, boiled, drained, diced (USDA)	1 cup	38	8.2
Frozen, Parmigiana (Buitoni)	4 oz.	189	16.2
Frozen, Parmigiana (Mrs. Paul's)	5½ oz.	250	21
Slices, frozen (Mrs. Paul's)	3 oz.	230	22
Sticks, frozen (Mrs. Paul's)	3½ oz.	260	27
Endive, Curly, including escarole (USDA)	2 oz.	10	2
Garlic, Raw, whole (USDA)	2 oz. (weighed with skin)	68	15.4
Raw, peeled (USDA)	1 oz.	39	8.7
Kale, Leaves, including stems, Cooked (USDA)	1 cup	30	4
Leeks, Raw, trimmed (USDA)	4 oz.	59	12.7
Lettuce, Butterhead as Boston types, head 4 in. diam. (USDA)	1 head	30	6
Crisp as Iceberg, 4-¾ in. diam. (USDA)	1 head	60	13
Looseleaf or bunching varieties, leaves (USDA)	2 large	10	2
Romaine, untrimmed (USDA)	1 lb.	52	10.2
Romaine, shredded & broken into pieces (USDA)	½ cup	4	.8
Mixed vegetables, Canned (Del Monte)	1 cup	80	16
Canned (Libby's)	1 cup	80	17
Frozen (Bird's Eye)	3.3 oz.	60	11
Frozen (Green Giant)	1 cup	90	16
In butter sauce, frozen (Mexicorn)	1 cup	130	17
Mushrooms, Canned (USDA)	1 cup	40	6
In butter sauce, frozen (Green Giant)	2 oz.	30	2
Whole, sliced, pieces and stems (Green Giant)	2 oz.	14	2
Mustard Greens, Chopped, frozen (Bird's Eye)	3.3 oz.	18	3

223

Food and Description	Measure or Quantity	Calories	Carbohydrates (grams)
Cooked (USDA)	1 cup	35	6
Okra, Cooked, pod 3 in. by 5/8 in. (USDA)	8 pods	25	5
Whole, frozen (Bird's Eye)	3.3 oz.	35	2
Onions, Boiled, Pearl onions (USDA)	½ cup	27	6.0
Boiled, whole (USDA)	1 cup	60	14
Canned, boiled, solids & liquid (Comstock-Greenwood)	4 oz.	33	7.4
Dehydrated, flakes (USDA)	1 cup	224	52.5
	1 tsp.	5	1.1
Frozen, chopped (Bird's Eye)	¼ cup	11	2.5
Frozen, small with cream sauce (Bird's Eye)	1/3 of pkg.	132	12.7
French-fried rings, canned, O-C (Durkee)	3½-oz. can	618	44.5
French-fried rings, frozen (Bird's Eye)	2 oz.	166	17.1
Mature, raw onion 2½ in. diam. (USDA)	1 onion	40	10
Onion rings, frozen (Mrs. Paul's)	2½ oz.	150	21
	5-oz. pkg.	418	41.3
	9-oz. pkg.	566	50.5
Raw, chopped (USDA)	1 tbsp.	4	1.0
	½ cup	33	7.5
Raw, grated (USDA)	1 tbsp.	5	1.2
Raw, slices (USDA)	½ cup	21	4.9
Raw, whole (USDA)	1 lb. (weighed untrimmed)	157	35.9
Small, creamed, frozen (Green Giant)	1 cup	100	16
	1/3 of 10-oz. pkg.	42	7.3
Small, whole, frozen (Bird's Eye)	4 oz.	40	9
Young green, small, without tops (USDA)	6 onions	20	5
Parsley, Fresh, chopped (USDA)	1 tbsp.	Trace	Trace
Fresh, whole (USDA)	½ lb.	100	19.3

Food and Description	Measure or Quantity	Calories	Carbohydrates (grams)
Parsnips, Cooked (USDA)	1 cup	100	23
Raw, whole (USDA)	1 lb. (weighed unpared)	293	67.5
Peas, Canned, solids & liquid (USDA)	1 cup	165	31
Early garden peas (Del Monte)	1 cup	110	20
Early peas with onions (Green Giant)	1 cup	120	22
Green, cooked (USDA)	1 cup	115	19
Green, immature, sweet (Libby's)	1 cup	120	23
Seasoned peas (Del Monte)	1 cup	120	25
Small early peas (Le Sueur)	1 cup	110	19
Small sweet peas (Le Sueur)	1 cup	100	17
Sweet (S & W Nutradiet)	½ cup	40	8
Sweet peas (Green Giant)	1 cup	110	17
Sweet, tiny size peas (Del Monte)	1 cup	100	18
Sweet peas with onions (Green Giant)	1 cup	110	17
Sweetlets, small sweet peas (Green Giant)	1 cup	100	17
Sweet green peas, frozen (Bird's Eye)	3.3 oz.	70	11
Sweet peas, frozen (Green Giant)	1 cup	100	16
Sweet peas in butter sauce, frozen (Le Sueur)	1 cup	150	18
Sweet peas in cream sauce (Le Sueur)	1 cup	160	25
Sweet peas with carrot points in cream sauce, frozen (Le Sueur)	1 cup	130	20
Sweet peas with onions in butter sauce, frozen (Le Sueur)	1 cup	140	16
Peas and Carrots (Del Monte)	1 cup	100	19
(Libby's)	1 cup	100	20

Food and Description	Measure or Quantity	Calories	Carbo-hydrates (grams)
(S & W Nutradiet)	½ cup	35	7
Dried Peas, Cowpeas or black-eye peas, dry, cooked (USDA)	1 cup	190	34
Peas, Split, Dry, cooked (USDA)	1 cup	290	52
Peppers, Sweet, green, raw, whole (USDA)	1 lb. (weighed untrimmed)	82	17.9
Sweet, raw, about 5 per lb., green pod without stem and seeds (USDA)	1 pod	15	4
Sweet, green raw, chopped (USDA)	½ cup	16	3.6
Sweet, green, raw, slices, (USDA)	½ cup	9	2.0
Sweet, green, raw, whole, without seeds and stems, strips (USDA)	½ cup (1.7 oz.)	11	2.4
Sweet, green, cooked, boiled, drained (USDA)	1 pod	15	3
Sweet, green, boiled, strips, drained (USDA)	½ cup	12	2.6
Sweet, red, raw, whole (USDA)	1 lb. (weighed with stems & seeds)	112	25.8
Sweet, red, raw, without stem and seeds (USDA)	1 med. pepper	19	2.4
Potatoes, French fried, frozen, heated (USDA)	10 pieces	125	19
French fried, 2 in. × ½ in. × ½ in., cooked in deep fat (USDA)	10 pieces	155	20
Medium, baked, peeled after baking (USDA)	1 potato	90	21
Medium, boiled, peeled after boiling (USDA)	1 potato	105	23

Food and Description	Measure or Quantity	Calories	Carbohydrates (grams)
Medium, peeled before boiling (USDA)	1 potato	80	18
New, canned (Del Monte)	1 cup	90	19
Mashed, milk added (USDA)	1 cup	125	25
Mashed, milk and butter added (USDA)	1 cup	185	24
Mashed flakes, Hungry Jack potatoes (Pillsbury)	½ cup	170	18
Potato Buds (Betty Crocker)	½ cup	60	14
Potatoes Au Gratin (Betty Crocker)	½ cup	90	19
Creamed (Betty Crocker)	½ cup	80	17
Hash browns with onions (Betty Crocker)	½ cup	90	20
Julienne (Betty Crocker)	½ cup	80	16
Scalloped (Betty Crocker)	½ cup	90	19
Sour cream 'n chive (Betty Crocker)	½ cup	90	17
Potato chips, medium, 2 in. diam. (USDA)	10 chips	115	10
Potato chips (Pringle)	1 oz.	150	16
Potatoes, Frozen, Baked, with cheese (Holloway House)	6 oz.	300	36
Baked, with sour cream (Holloway House)	6 oz.	280	36
Bake-A-Tata with cheese (Holloway House)	5 oz.	220	27
Bake-A-Tata with sour cream (Holloway House)	5 oz.	200	27
Potatoes Au Gratin casserole (Green Giant)	1 cup	250	38
Potatoes Romanoff casserole (Green Giant)	1 cup	250	35
Scalloped potatoes casserole (Green Giant)	1 cup	240	40
Pumpkin, Canned (Del Monte)	1 cup	80	18
Canned (Libby's)	1 cup	80	20
Radishes, Small, raw, without tops (USDA)	4 radishes	5	Trace

227

Food and Description	Measure or Quantity	Calories	Carbo-hydrates (grams)
Rutabaga, Boiled, diced, drained (USDA)	½ cup	30	7.1
Boiled, mashed (USDA)	½ cup	43	10.0
Canned (King Pharr)	½ cup	52	
Raw, diced (USDA)	½ cup	32	7.7
Raw, without tops (USDA)	1 lb. (weighed with skin)	177	42.4
Sauerkraut, Canned (Del Monte)	1 cup	50	11
Canned (Libby's)	1 cup	40	10
Canned, solids & liquid (USDA)	1 cup	45	9
Spinach, Canned (Del Monte)	1 cup	45	7
Canned (Libby's)	1 cup	45	7
Canned, drained solids (USDA)	1 cup	45	6
Cooked (USDA)	1 cup	40	6
Creamed, frozen (Bird's Eye)	3 oz.	60	6
Creamed, frozen (Le Sueur)	1 cup	140	11
In butter sauce, frozen (Le Sueur)	1 cup	90	6
Deviled spinach casserole, frozen (Green Giant)	1 cup	160	11
Squash, Summer, Cooked, diced (USDA)	1 cup	30	7
Crookneck & Straightneck, fresh, yellow, whole (USDA)	1 lb. (weighed untrimmed)	89	19.1
Crookneck & Straightneck, fresh, yellow, boiled, drained, sliced (USDA)	½ cup	13	2.7
Scallop, fresh, white & pale green, whole (USDA)	1 lb. (weighed untrimmed)	93	22.7
Scallop, fresh, white & pale green, boiled, drained, mashed (USDA)	½ cup	19	4.5

Food and Description	Measure or Quantity	Calories	Carbohydrates (grams)
Zucchini & Cocozelle, fresh, green, whole *(USDA)*	1 lb. (weighed untrimmed)	73	15.5
Zucchini & Cocozelle, fresh, green, boiled, drained slices *(USDA)*	½ cup	9	1.9
Zucchini in tomato sauce, canned *(Del Monte)*	½ cup	25	5.6
Frozen, not thawed *(USDA)*	4 oz.	24	5.3
Frozen, boiled, drained *(USDA)*	4 oz.	24	5.3
Frozen, fried, breaded, zucchini *(Mrs. Paul's)*	9-oz. pkg.	566	62.5
Frozen, parmesan, zucchini *(Mrs. Paul's)*	12-oz. pkg.	259	16.0
Frozen, slices *(Bird's Eye)*	½ cup	20	3.8
Frozen, zucchini *(Bird's Eye)*	1/3 pkg.	20	2.3
Squash, Winter, Acorn, fresh, whole *(USDA)*	1 lb. (weighed with skin & seeds)	152	38.6
Acorn, baked, flesh only *(USDA)*	1 cup	130	32
Acorn, fresh, flesh only, boiled, mashed *(USDA)*	½ cup	39	9.7
Butternut, fresh, whole *(USDA)*	1 lb. (weighed with skin & seeds)	171	44.4
Butternut, fresh, baked, flesh only *(USDA)*	4 oz.	77	19.8
Butternut, fresh, boiled, flesh only *(USDA)*	4 oz.	46	11.8
Hubbard, fresh, whole *(USDA)*	1 lb. (weighed	117	28.1

Food and Description	Measure or Quantity	Calories	Carbohydrates (grams)
	with skin & seeds)		
Hubbard, fresh, baked, flesh only (USDA)	4 oz.	57	13.3
Hubbard, fresh, baked, flesh only, mashed (USDA)	½ cup	51	11.9
Hubbard, fresh, boiled, flesh only, diced (USDA)	½ cup	35	8.1
Hubbard, fresh, boiled, flesh only, mashed (USDA)	½ cup	37	8.4
Frozen, not thawed (USDA)	4 oz.	43	10.4
Frozen, heated (USDA)	½ cup	46	11.0
Frozen (Bird's Eye)	4 oz.	95	1.7
Succotash, Cream style, canned (Libby's)	1 cup	190	45
Whole kernel, canned (Libby's)	1 cup	150	35
Frozen (Bird's Eye)	3.3 oz.	80	17
Sweet potatoes, Baked, medium, peeled after baking (USDA)	1 potato	155	36
Boiled, peeled after boiling (USDA)	1 potato	170	39
Candied (USDA)	1 potato	295	60
Canned (USDA)	1 cup	235	54
Tomatoes, Canned, solids & liquid (USDA)	1 cup	50	10
Raw, approx. 3 in. diam., 2-1/8 in. high, wt. 7 oz. (USDA)	1 tomato	40	9
Stewed, canned (Contadina)	1 cup	70	18
Stewed, canned (Del Monte)	1 cup	70	16
Stewed, canned (Hunt-Wesson)	4 oz.	30	7
Stewed, canned (Libby's)	1 cup	60	15
Tomato Wedges, canned (Del Monte)	1 cup	60	14
Whole peeled, canned (Contadina)	1 cup	50	11

Food and Description	Measure or Quantity	Calories	Carbohydrates (grams)
Whole, peeled, canned (Del Monte)	1 cup	50	10
Whole peeled, canned (Hunt-Wesson)	4 oz.	20	5
Whole peeled, canned (Libby's)	1 cup	45	10
Whole, canned (S & W Nutra diet)	½ cup	25	5
Turnips, Cooked, diced (USDA)	1 cup	35	8
Chopped turnip greens, frozen (Bird's Eye)	3.3 oz.	20	2
Chopped turnip greens with diced turnips, frozen (Bird's Eye)	3.3 oz.	20	3
Turnip greens, cooked (USDA)	1 cup	30	5

S
V

NOTES

NOTES

NOTES

NOTES

NOTES

NOTES

NOTES